LATE FRAGMENT

Notes on the
Later Stages of Life

Dr. Charles H. Edwards II

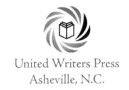

United Writers Press
Asheville, N.C.

ISBN: 978-1-952248-52-8 (print)
ISBN: 978-1-952248-53-5 (ebook)

Published by:
United Writers Press
Asheville, N.C.
www.uwpnew.com

Artwork by
Leslie Edwards

Sales from this book support
Memory & Movement Charlotte
www.mmclt.org

Printed in the U.S.A.

For Mary

*"She wasn't doing a thing that I could see
except standing there, leaning on the balcony
railing, holding the universe together."*

— J.D. Salinger, "A Girl I Knew"

Contents

Author's Note / Acknowledgments

Following the Introduction, the book is divided into three parts. Part 1, Background, is where we define in sequence the time period under discussion and who is in the *late fragment*. It is crucial that we do so.

The book is a complicated study of the last stage of human life and the thoughts, fears, hopes and behavior of those humans living in it. Most of the takeaways and insights that define this time are not relevant to earlier stages of lives. They will not resonate or seem understandable if this fact is overlooked. Part 2, Jeopardy, is the hard part. This is where the dangers, toils and snares are named and exposed. It is a necessary on-ramp to Part 3, Directive. The final chapters are emotional, strategic maps meant to guide us to relevance, calm and purpose as we approach the uncharted environs that are certainties in long lives.

I suggest you read each chapter as a singular unit and process it alone. We are confronting the basic elements of aging. Loss, decline, loneliness and survival are only the beginning. The book is intended to project you into a myriad of situations so that you can benefit from the challenges of others or recognize yourself in a story or profile. I hope these confrontations provide insight and a deeper understanding of what humans need as they near life's end.

The stories are all true. The individuals profiled have lived and exhibited the behaviors described. In some instances, personal details have been changed to honor the privacy of those individuals. These details occurred but to a different person or at a different time. All individuals still living have given permission for their story to be shared in the context intended.

The interviews and dialogue are as close to factual as memory allows. In each conversation, my comments are preceded with my initials, CHE. My interview style and bedside manner have been described as direct, bold and, on occasion, audacious. I take those descriptions as compliments.

I have numerous individuals to thank.

I owe an enormous debt of gratitude to everyone who allowed me to talk to them about their lives. They shared what worked and were willing to share what didn't. That took courage. Many of these individuals are gone. I hope the stories they shared are a fitting legacy for their lives.

Hannah Barnes, a recent graduate of Cornell University and a two-summer intern at Memory & Movement Charlotte, researched multiple topics and helped with the bibliography.

Again, my editor and friend, Ken Garfield, was instrumental from the beginning. He convinced me that this book needed to be written and provided guidance and valuable criticism throughout the process.

I also want to acknowledge contributions from Vally Sharpe at United Writers Press in Asheville, N.C. She helped us with both *Late Fragment* and *Much Abides* and sheds light exactly where it is needed.

I owe special thanks to my daughter Leslie and son Chuck for their time and talents. Their contributions not only made the book infinitely better but enormous fun. Leslie did all the art. Her eye for the world and her paintbrush transfer love and understanding to everything she sees or touches. Chuck, with his light and enlightened approach, rescued me from the depths of writer's block and reignited the passion I had for this subject when I thought it was gone.

And finally thanks to Mary, who simply holds OUR universe together.

Charles H Edwards II
October 2023

"This *late fragment,* our last act,
has the potential to be the best of times. But it is tricky."

Chuck Edwards

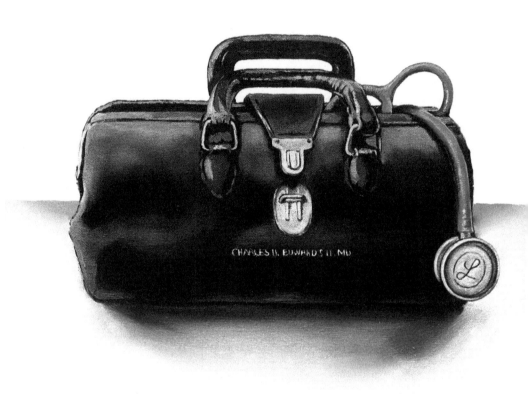

Introduction

This book is a sequel to a book I wrote in 2020 entitled *Much Abides: A Survival Guide for Aging Lives.*[1] My purpose in writing that book was to make individuals aware of the natural effects of aging on our brains and how those effects alter our perceptions and behavior. It primarily focused on the transition from career to retirement. The goal was to improve our chances of making the later stages of life joyful and relevant by identifying the factors that either enhanced or undermined the chances of achieving that goal.

This book has the same goal but its focus is a later interval. I call this the *late fragment*, the time closer to the end.

The idea for the book began soon after the first book was published. I was invited to speak about the book at a retirement center here in my hometown of Charlotte, N.C. I knew this audience well. This would be a mix of longtime friends, medical colleagues and patients. Some of the patients would be from my first career as a cardiovascular surgeon. Others would be patients of my current practice, Memory & Movement Charlotte, caring for patients with dementia and those who care for them. I would look forward to seeing these individuals and sharing the bond that only a surgeon who had operated on them more than thirty years ago or a physician who is involved with the daily struggle against memory loss would understand.

As I was preparing the talk, I realized that this group was beyond the scope of *Much Abides*, long past the transition from career to retirement. When I projected forward and looked into the faces of my prospective audience, I saw individuals in their mid- to late-80s and early 90s, whose lives had new, urgent concerns. The reality of these lives were limits forced on them by age. Those limits differed from person to person, some physical, some mental. Losses varied from simple effects of aging—slowing in thought and action, mobility challenges—to devastating health issues—strokes, heart failure, etc. The most devastating were losses of a spouse or an adult child. At least half were now caregivers for a spouse, which meant they not only had their own limits but had to deal with the accelerated and relentless decline of someone they loved. The loss of mobility was often matched by a decline in will.

I became aware of common threads in each of these groups. The limitations altered their passion for life, their view of the future and relationships with family and friends. This phase and the people in it deserved a deeper look. If the time with this group was going to have value for them, I was going to have to change my focus. I was being forced into a later period in their lives. This was past second careers. For many, it was beyond travel and even beyond volunteering. If I had any hope of saying anything worthwhile, I would need to learn more. What are their lives really like when we pull off the social masks? Do they still have hope to match fear? What are the expectations of every day?

I started from scratch. My goal was to learn as much as possible about the lives of those faces in the audience. I did literature searches, read extensively and interviewed multiple men and women actually living in the late phase. This, combined with the daily experience of caring for this age group in my medical practice, allowed me to see a profile emerge of what possibilities lay ahead, what worked and what didn't. The upside was unique to the individual, each having their own answers to the questions at hand. The downside, the despair, looked the same in everyone that had it.

In the early going, the upside was compelling. I had selected individuals who at least on the surface were navigating successfully these late years. Looking back, I had selected a profile that appeared to have this end game figured out. The questions I asked and the answers received fit the profile and created a bias.

But this select group of successful portraits didn't tell the full story. I wanted to identify the positives, but I needed to see the struggles more clearly. When I started asking the right questions, a different story, more complex and often troubling, emerged.

Two shadows came over the process which forced me to stop writing and to question whether I even wanted to write this book. The first shadow was the reality of lives in the last years. Yes, some flourished, but many did not. The stories were complicated and patterns of loneliness, loss and despair were common. Even the individuals who claimed that "this is a great time in my life," when reexamined admitted to profound challenges. To make the effort to understand the complicated and layered factors controlling these late effects, there had to be a payoff. Some strategies would have to evolve from the effort to potentially offset the downside of this project and actually identify themes, habits and truths that could function as grab bars or sources of light to safely guide individuals through these fragile and scary times.

The second shadow fell on me. When I was writing about "them," these old people, it was easy to make observations in the search for hope at this stage of life. The weight of the reality of aging opened my eyes to the fact that this was possibly my future. Do I really want to struggle with these demons now? Why not live with the illusion that it will never come and, when it does, deal with it? Maybe I will be spared, struck by lightning just before a late decline. Does projecting ourselves into future phases of life have the potential to help us avoid major pitfalls and possibly outrun despair?

The answer is YES. But the process is fraught with anxiety, the loss of illusions, and requires smashing into painful facts. The process, if done fearlessly, has the potential to awaken a calmness and joy for life that we have longed for our entire adult lives.

I have spent the last two years living daily with the individuals in the *late fragment*. Their lives have dominated my thoughts. I know these individuals, what they fear, what they hope. I know what questions to ask and what their answers mean. I have an instinct for any neglect, loneliness or despair. I have been educated in what works and what makes it work. What started out as an arm's length, semi-intellectual pursuit to better understand my patients and their caregivers has ended in an intense, almost suffocating, personal trek to understand the deeper meanings of life.

I have two aspirations for the book.

First, that all involved, the children, families, colleagues and people next door, will understand the challenges faced by my soulmates in the late stages of life. I want those aging individuals to be approached with honor for the lives they have led. I want this understanding and respect to lead to the development of strategies to ensure that the time left is dignified and, if possible, enjoyable.

Second, that the individuals who are living close to the end don't give up. I want them to find new, clever ways to remain vital. They still know things we need to know.

As in other times in my life, what I expected was not what I got. But what I got was far better than what I expected. I was thrown off course early when the search took me to some unexpected dark places. I worried that there would not be enough resolve, enough hope to justify the search. I have never been more wrong in my life. The more individuals I interviewed, listened to and befriended, the more I realized the courage, resolve and tenacity in these individuals was more than a match for the challenges of living a long time. We are going to cover these challenges in depth and offer soft suggestions and directions for meeting and overcoming them.

Most importantly, I need your trust that I would never have started this book unless I thought I could deliver on the promise of making this *late fragment* of life not just tolerable but worthy of the lives that preceded.

This will be a wild ride. Hold on.

LATE FRAGMENT

Part I
Background

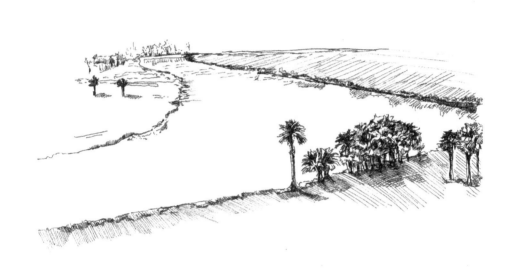

1

Age and Culture

The place in which I'll fit will not exist until I make it.

James Baldwin

There is a story, perhaps apocryphal, about a Bedouin tribe and how each year they come face to face with death.[1] The tribe lives at a subsistence level which requires them to seek out higher, more fertile grasslands for their flock of sheep in the summer. The tribe depends on the sheep and their vitality to survive. To do this, they have to cross a wide, dangerous river late in the spring to get to the higher meadows. Each member of the tribe must be able to cross the river independently, which makes this the breakpoint for the aged. The tribe cannot risk losing one of their strong leaders by helping older members across.

The culture of the tribe is well established. All members are aware of the peril the river presents each year. The very old will not attempt to cross and are left on the bank to die. All but the oldest attempt to cross but risk being swept downstream. One can only imagine how heartbreaking it would be to leave one's mother or father on the bank knowing you are sentencing them to certain death.

This is obviously a stark, abrupt approach on the part of one tribe to deal with aging and death. It is a stretch to think that this drama at the riverbank, with its distance from us in circumstance, time and culture, could guide us in any way. Actually that stretch is worth a closer look.

Valuable lessons and unexpected connections often come from the far edges of our experience. This became clear to me when I began caring for patients with dementia. The pathological process of aging that we term dementia is often nothing more than an exaggerated version of normal aging. Often, witnessing and understanding these exaggerations help us understand our own predicaments, the dangers and even the values that are less obvious but present.

The Bedouin anguish at the riverbank serves that purpose. If you strip away the shock and the unnerving visual, it is one way of doing it. Let me explain.

Every society, every tribe, must address the basics of life for a specific group of humans. How and what they decide establishes the uniqueness of their bonds to one another. The process addresses who will lead them, what values those leaders will have and how they will be selected. It will include the distinct roles of men and women, the raising of children, access to food and whether they will be peaceful or warlike. The taboos around sex, birth and death will be central to their unique culture.

A major concern in all societies is the value of aging individuals. What do we do with the elders who once led, contributed and sacrificed and now can no longer pull their weight? Are they valued for their past contributions and sought out for their wisdom or perceived as a burden and tolerated but not cherished?

Do cultures that cherish aging members have advantages over societies that dismiss their value? It would seem that groups of individuals who value the aged would be more secure and predictable. If a young man knows that he will be respected until he dies, he will sacrifice for others. If he knows that his hour of respect and influence is short-lived, he is more likely to be anxious, selfish and bellicose. If a young woman sees older women being valued for their roles of providing for the tribe and raising children, she will play that role with reverence. The husbands and children will predictably be more secure and connected to the values of the tribe.

How the elders perceive themselves and their late-in-life roles will be a crucial factor in the temper of the tribe. If they are the recipients of love and respect, they will assume new roles. These roles are less active but just as important. The role of teacher and the transferring of character traits from one generation to the next is the vital link to developing future leaders.

Back to the Bedouins. I don't know why this ritual at the river has stuck with me. Initially it was the scene of anguish at the riverbank, thinking of leaving someone I love to certain, immediate death.

Morbidly, I wondered what those left behind would do. Would they lie down and give up or struggle in some way? I just couldn't see it. I could hear my mother yelling, "Chuck Edwards, don't you dare leave me!" But that's another story.

The Bedouins have two lessons to pass on. Both stem from their distinct ties to death.

The first is the scene at the end of a life. Modern medicine has delivered on the promise of healthier, longer lives. We are fortunate to have this benefit that is so consequential in our lives.

Sadly, there is a time when the inevitable is certain, fixed. If the hope for miracles is carried too far, it prevents the final scene from unfolding. The insistence that "this is not over" forces all involved to instead foster an illusion, a false agenda. Both the departing and those who will live on are hurt by this. Those at the end of their lives never get to play out the final scene, to experience those important words, hugs and feelings that all of us want at the end. For those who will go on living, the false agenda prevents closure and the accompanying reverence that is vital to their coming to peace with it all. Often, regrets are the legacy.

There may be regrets on the riverbank for the Bedouins, but it is not from any illusion that "this is not over" or "I am not prepared." This late drama has been hardwired into their existence from the beginning. They have said goodbye to people they love on this spot many times. There is no possibility that the enormity and significance of what is unfolding will be lost or misunderstood.

That is Lesson No. 1. If you are going or staying, pay attention! It matters.

The second lesson is made clear in a late image I have of the riverbank. There is an old man approaching the river. He sees the current raging in front of him. He knows he is on his own. He has left his grandparents and his parents on the bank of this river. Again, he knows the drill. His feelings are of resolve and defiance rather than surrender. There is boldness in his thoughts—"I would rather drown in this river, right here, right now, then weakly wait out a fate on the riverbank."

He enters the river with slow, careful steps. He is immediately overcome by the current and must walk, swim and panic his way across. He emerges on the other side, choking on and throwing up silty river water. He rolls over on his back to look at the sun to convince himself that he has made it across. That he is still alive.

His first thoughts are, "It was a miracle I made it. The fates delivered me, maybe for a purpose."

The thought that follows is, "I have an entire year before I have to do that again. I am going to make it a good one." The brave Bedouin has a valuable lesson to share. The awareness that time is limited makes the time left more precious.

I have covered this concept early because it is a necessary step in understanding and navigating the *late fragment* of life. We don't have to be consumed by the thought of dying. But we should carry the realization that this play will eventually close.

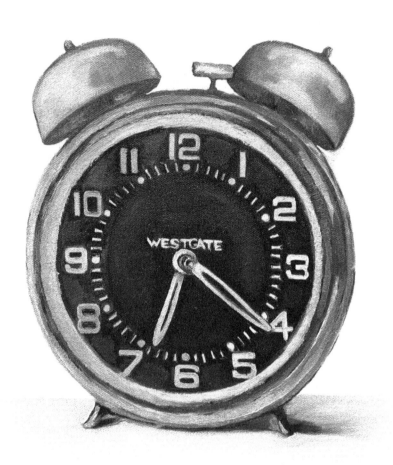

2
A Gift of Time?

I am going to define the *late fragment* as the time in life that follows everything that is supposedly significant. It is past career, past active retirement, past travel, past volunteering. There will be important events in life but they will involve members of one's family—graduations, weddings, the birth of a grandchild or great- grandchild. With the exception of a late birthday or possibly anniversary, seemingly nothing major is ahead for you. Oh wait. There is one, final, monumental event...your own death.

What purpose beyond wanting to shock could be served by that sentence? My purpose is to alert you, warn may be a better word, that what follows is serious business. There is tough, anxiety-producing stuff ahead. It also starkly defines the limits of the time in life we plan to cover.

Last and most importantly, it introduces the reality into this final chapter of life, that accepting the inevitability of one's death and allowing it to change our perception of time is crucial to making these late hours precious.

But I am getting ahead of myself again. Let's start with a hard look at this "gift of time."

Americans are living longer. The average life span of a female today is just shy of 80 years. In 2050, it is estimated there will be 400,000 individuals over 100. That number today is circa 80,000. Surely this is a gift that modern science bestows on those living in this era. Healthier lives, more time.[1,2]

But there's a catch. When will we experience this benefit of time? Will I spend more time in school? Will I get more than four years in college? Will my children be with me longer? The answer is a resounding NO.

Careers may be marginally longer. Early retirement may be longer and more active because of modern health benefits. Sadly, though, the majority of this overtime will come late. If one survives long enough, fortunate to avoid disease and catastrophe, the benefit will be tacked on to the end of life. A *late fragment*.

Navigating the end game, making those late years joyful, connected and even productive, will require perspective and skills that are not needed when we occupied the corridors of power.

Success requires sacrifice. What am I willing to give up in order to play this game of life? In school, in sports, in careers, certain attributes are rewarded. Some are not. Dedication to the task, singularity of purpose, willingness to delay gratification are rewarded. Listening to your own drummer, living life on your terms and stopping to smell the roses, not so much.

Each of us has repeated this process throughout our lives. We search the potential of each phase of life and actively scan for what is achievable. We then roll the dice, matching our wits and talents against the system. We are pre-programmed for these steps. We have repeated the process countless times for every big decision. What activities do I want to pursue? What college? What spouse? What career? When to retire? Where? There is always a future with new and exciting goals. There is always the fallback that if I veer off, there is time to adjust, to get it right after all.

This process lets us down later in life. We find ourselves in a space where the words *future* and *time* take on new meaning, often overshadowed by uncertainty. The attributes we relied on earlier in our life no longer assure even a sliver of success. Somebody somewhere has moved the goalpost, altered the rules of the game. It actually is worse than that. It is not even the same game.

Please note. My intent is not to scare but to create tension to emphasize the stakes that are in play. The negative consequences of the illusion that life flows on without major shifts in perspective and behavior is more confounding and potentially crippling the longer you hold on to it. This *late fragment*, our last act, has the potential to be the best of times. But it is tricky. Fundamental shifts in expectations are required to pull it off.

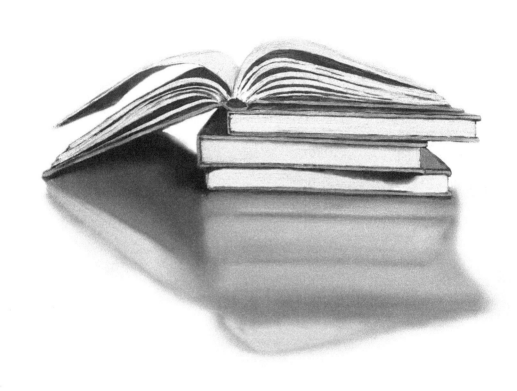

3

Even So

It is difficult to get the news from poems, yet men die
miserably every day for lack of what is found there.

William Carlos Williams

And did you get what you wanted from this life, even so?
I did.
And what did you want?
To call myself beloved, to feel
myself beloved on this earth.
— *Raymond Carver, "Late Fragment"*

When he wrote the poem, "Late Fragment," Raymond Carver was dying of cancer at age 50. The poem, inscribed on his tombstone, would be the last thing he would write for publication.[1]

He is known for the simple, direct and sometimes raw use of words in his short stories and poems. He relished being a solo character, disarmingly unapologetic for what he thought and wrote.[2,3]

Incapable of anything short of staring down his fate without pity or panic, simply accepting what he had wrought.

The poem asks two questions and provides two answers: Did you get what you wanted from life? And what did you want? Simple, direct. At the end of the first question, he adds the words "even so."

Even so. Almost slang. But the words take on a deep meaning. This is the final tally of all the minuses and pluses of a life. Even so, was this a life worth living? In the end, did you get what you wanted? He answers "I did." This is a man who had demons to the point that he tried to kill himself with alcohol by the age of 40. No shortage of minuses here.

In the answer to the second question, he explains how he can make that claim in the face of a lifetime of woes. What is it you wanted? He tells us that by being able to call himself beloved and to feel beloved, the scales tip toward this being all worth it.

Each of us will have a different take on what it means to be beloved. It may involve family, lifelong bonds that connect generations with love and concern. It may involve connections to colleagues with whom a mentor role was mutually affirming or to one person who proved central to everything valuable in one's life. Whatever the bond, I can assure you that it involves human beings. The tethering to others is the source of authentic value and joy in every human life. Those who miss this fact risk a frightening isolation as lives move toward the end. Possessions, financial success and prestige cannot sustain one late. A consistent theme in all the interviews and interactions

I conducted was that isolation and loneliness are precursors to anxiety, despair and, tragically, panic as the end nears.

The deeper I went into the lives of those in the *late fragment*, the more I found this link to other humans uniquely irreplaceable.

Raymond Carver's final words said as much.

I have entitled this book *Late Fragment*. It fits. The word fragment describes this late stage in all our lives. Bits and shreds of joy and purpose intertwined with decline, loss and uncertainty. How do we keep our balance in such uneven, unpredictable environs?

We have started by defining the time period and the stakes involved. We have emphasized the demands that this late phase forces and how crucial those adjustments are to the final outcome. One can be impressively successful in every former stage of one's life but falter late, finishing bitter and emotionally starved. We are about to set off on an odyssey to prevent that outcome.

The ultimate goal of the journey is to prepare us for those final moments when the fates tap us on the shoulder and say, "It's time."

As we turn away, they ask, "Did you get what you wanted out of this life?"

You have prepared for this moment. The answer is, "Even so, I did."

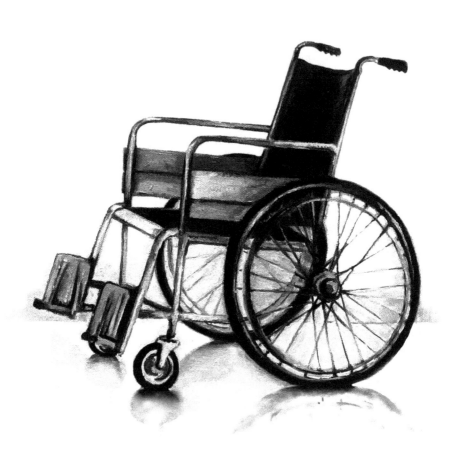

4

Who's In?

Sharon Murdock is the wife of a colleague of mine. I have known her for 40 years. I had not seen her for several years following a move with her husband to Texas to be closer to their children and grandchildren. They returned to Charlotte for a visit. We had dinner with Sharon and her husband, Michael. Our families were close for years with our children being the same ages and attending the same school. At dinner, I was eager to learn the fate of her father. He was a physician at the end of his career when mine was just beginning. I enjoyed his company and his take on medicine and life.

CHE: Sharon, how is your dad? I hope he is doing OK.

Sharon: Chuck, he died last year at 95. It could not have been harder at the end.

CHE: I'm sorry to hear that. I was always impressed by his zeal for life. He seemed to enjoy all his roles—physician, dad and granddad. He was at all the games. I loved hearing him good-naturedly taunt referees. I hope he got to play golf until the end. No one loved golf more than he did.

Sharon: Chuck, you are nice to remember those times. I have forgotten most of them. This may sound harsh and insensitive but the last 10 years were so bad that I have a hard time even remembering the good times. If he could have died at 85, he would be revered at this point. But he lived to 95. I apologize for dumping this on you, but I am struggling with the thought of enduring 10 years of his torment and anger, most of it directed at me. He thought I could fix the effects of age and the loss of not only my mother but his physical decline. He had all his marbles until the end but died a selfish, bitter man. Up to 85, life had been a triumph. He was a great dad, husband and grandfather. I wish he had been struck by lightning at 85. He was great on the up but couldn't handle the down.

It has affected me. I am now fearful that I could turn into that bitter and frustrated person when I get to that stage of life. I don't want my kids to have the feelings toward me that I have toward my father. My children even now avoid talking about him. Let's talk about something else. This is too hard.

This conversation was more than two years ago, but it struck a deep, sorrowful chord. A man lives 85 years of his life enjoying vital and warm connections to family and friends. He is fortunate on one hand to live another 10 years but is unable to sustain the role that fostered those endearing relationships. The last act is tragic. For whatever reason, he is unable to adjust to the loss and decline inherent in the late phase of long lives.

The legacy is painful—recent memories of hard times, not decades of good times.

The *late fragment* will exact its due. If approached with the knowledge that new approaches and perspective will be needed to stay connected, it has the potential to give joy and purpose to the end.

Part 2 of the book is a quest to examine every challenge, pitfall and sinkhole that has the potential to thwart our desire to flourish late. The first step is to understand the fundamentals of the *late fragment*.

Let's start with who is in this stage and why.

Who's In?

Group I: Healthy old people. Lots of them.

The largest group in the *late fragment* results from age alone. You live long enough, you get a bid. Decline is built into the system.

The obvious declines are physical. They are seen and felt. They are inescapable. One can outrun them for a stretch. But the longer you are in the game, the more certain the encounters. What is seen are the cosmetic effects of aging. The facial signs jump off the surface of the mirror to the point that we sometimes wonder if we are looking at a stranger. The slowing of reflexes and gait. The subtle signs of imbalance. Arthritic changes in the spine, hands and feet.

What is felt is the slowness in reaction, stiffness in joints, decline in strength and exaggerated soreness following exercise.

The gradual loss of balance is an actual metaphor for this process of growing old. These changes are all predictable and should be expected.

There is a simple way to avoid these late-life insults. But that solution has its own downside. It involves dying before the effects of age get started. I'll take the wrinkles and stiffness.

If we live long enough, we are forced to deal with the effects of time on our bodies and minds. The question is, "What does 'deal with them' mean?" Does it mean fight against the decline? Yes. Does it mean doing everything in your power to minimize the damage? Absolutely. Does denying that they are occurring or resenting the results have a place? No.

How we respond is the key to remaining vital and relevant in these later stages. One of the universal goals is to live a long, healthy life. When that happens, we cannot undermine the satisfaction of having made it by being bitter and angry over the compromises inherent in the process. This is Group I. Lots of older individuals experiencing normal physical and cognitive aging.

Group II: Individuals with disabilities.

The longer we live, the greater the percentage of individuals living with a disability. This group is divided into two distinct tiers, those whose disability occurred early in their lives and those that occurred late.

The individuals who were born with challenges or developed challenges early in life don't need a blueprint for navigating any phase in life. They have passed that test. They have accepted the fact that life is a daily challenge and are used to making compromises to survive. They will enter the *late fragment* at some point, often younger than their contemporaries. I write this paragraph only to make the rest of us aware that when age is superimposed on those special needs, we must pay attention. A helping hand may be needed to complement the strength that has always been there.

The second tier, those who have suffered late injuries and medical illness, face major obstacles. I include those who are disabled from strokes, falls, crippling arthritis and the like. I also include cardiac, pulmonary and the myriad of chronic diseases. I exclude those with terminal illnesses. They are in a different setting and a separate group.

There is a common thread in these individuals. It is a lack of mobility. Patients with strokes, Parkinson's or an injury from a fall or arthritis have physical limits to movement. An individual who earlier in life moved effortlessly and purposefully, who now is trapped in a body that makes even simple adjustments a struggle, presents a larger test to stay relevant. There is also the stigma, evident to all, that "I am impaired." The obvious deficits left by a stroke or the impaired gait of a patient with Parkinson's often result in embarrassment and self-imposed isolation. A major goal of families, friends and those caring for these individuals is convincing them of their value and importance despite the change in physical fortunes.

Those with systemic illnesses involving the heart and lungs, chronic malignancies and the like also contend with mobility but in a different way. Fatigue is the limiting factor. Many of us who contracted COVID 19 got a glimpse of the debilitation that fatigue unleashes on otherwise normal individuals. Simply walking across a room resulted in breathlessness and anxiety. Imagine the psychological trauma if this weariness was permanent. To have a positive impact on these two subgroups, we must start with strategies to help them MOVE. They are trapped in bodies that no longer can reliably transport them to centers of activity. Being aware of this and adapting strategies to overcome it will allow the physical impairment to be minimized and the person's presence and relevance preserved.

That is Group II. Smaller numbers than Group I but demanding more compassion and energy to make this somehow work.

Group III: Patients with dementia.

I am including these individuals in a separate category because of the unique nature of the disease that afflicts them. Loss of memory and cognitive decline has resulted in their losing their voice and impact in life. Except for Mild Cognitive Impairment and early dementia, the potential to change the course of the disease is limited. We can make the patients calm, safe, clean and loved. But the disease itself has resisted every attempt to reverse its effect. We don't even know what causes it.

I often make the point that there is a time in each of these patient's illness that marks a profound change in our approach. We go from being in the memory business to being in the dignity business. Evidence of this priority shift is on every wall and shelf in our clinic, where paintings and artwork done by our patients are displayed. In my office, I have a shelf of books authored by our patients. A prized possession is a carving of a duck, a decoy, by an artist known throughout the world for his carvings. We display these treasures for three reasons. 1) New patients who enter will see them and realize they, too, will be valued and their contributions noted. 2) Families are aware that patients have been diminished and their voices hushed. Society and its stigma of memory loss and psychiatric illness has written them off. We always ask for details about the patient, about their careers and interests. These questions about the patient and family, and featuring patients' art on the walls, symbolize to the world that HERE in our clinic they are not written off. I also want all involved to realize that as long as we are in business, they will live forever on these walls. 3) The final reason is for all of us who work at Memory & Movement Charlotte. It reminds us that these patients have had dignified lives. They have accomplished amazing things. It is our job to treat them with dignity and, in the end, get them out of this world with that dignity intact.

That is Group III. For us, it is a large group. For the world, though, it is a small and diminished band. It is our role to remind the world of their impact and to speak for them.

Group IV: Those at the very end.

As I mentioned in earlier chapters, I spend a great deal of time with patients who have reached the end. This is the period at the end of a long, painful sentence. It is time. I am not sad. If the family is assembled, attentive and calm, I have done my job.

My hope is always that the family will be closer, more understanding of one another. That the illness, this unrelenting, pitiless disease, will have healed fault lines in families forever.

The love that comes out of this turmoil and travail has the power to heal, sustain and elevate lives. It is there at the bedside, the last gift from the soul turning away from us and toward their lot. It is always my wish that the hole left by the departing one will be filled with greater tolerance and love between the survivors.

That is Group IV.

Groups I, II, III and IV share a common thread—they increasingly depend on caregivers. I had originally planned to present caregivers as Group V but it does not do them the justice they deserve. They are chronologically not yet in the *late fragment*, but they are living through it. Understanding their roles in aging lives and their indispensable impact on the success of those who are actually in the *late fragment* requires a deeper, more respectful breakdown.

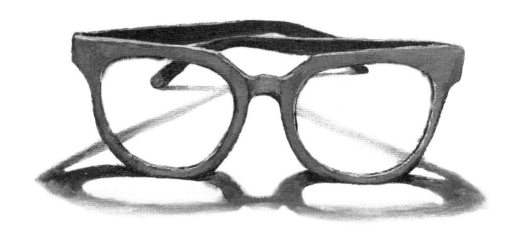

5
Limits of Devotion

There are only four kinds of people in the world—those who have been caregivers, those who are currently caregivers, those who will be caregivers and those who will need caregivers.

Rosalynn Carter in her testimony before
the Senate Special Committee on Aging, May 26, 2011.

During the four months I spent at Johns Hopkins University learning to care for patients with dementia, the patient was the primary focus. What were the presenting symptoms? Did they have behavioral issues? What stage were they in? What medications might help? My focus was entirely on the patient and the disease.

When I returned to Charlotte, it became clear immediately that I could not help the patient if I didn't help the caregiver. As the disease progresses, our focus shifts more to the caregiver. Finally, at the end and even after, the caregiver is central.

Caregivers are all in the *late fragment*. The demands of the individuals they care for dominate their lives. The personal dreams and desires of their lives have been put on hold. No matter how sincere the effort or how effective the strategies, the demands increase. Watching someone you love struggle and decline causes emotional exhaustion and physical fatigue. The potential for guilt and despair is always near.

Having framed the caregiver experience in this difficult light, one would be astonished at how often it is done with dedication and profound self-sacrifice. Each caregiver situation is unique. It starts long before there is a need for a caregiver. The relationship that precedes the illness sets the stage and establishes the depth and strength of the bonds that are tested by age and decline. Each caregiver is tested in their own way. Their response to those demands are unique to them.

I am going to share two caregiver scenarios that cover very different situations. You are in line to meet three resourceful, unbreakable ladies whose stories provide insights and strategies applicable to every caregiver situation.

The Sandwich: A Double Decker

Anne Decker is 75 years old. She is principal caregiver for her husband, Clint. He is 80 and has been having memory and cognitive issues for four years. He now is asking repetitive questions and exhibiting rapid forgetting. He has lost multiple credit cards and sets of keys. He has gotten lost while driving even in familiar surroundings. Clint can no longer solve simple problems. He is no longer able to balance a checkbook or manage his finances, both strengths in the past. A common phenomenon at this stage is obsessions, often with money. He insists on carrying large amounts of cash and displaying it, making him a target for harm.

The patient is a proud man. He is the first in his family to graduate from college, which preceded a successful stint in the Air Force. He was proud of his 30-year career with an airline and carried his awards and citations with him to medical office visits. The patient has no insight into his memory challenges, which makes caring for him difficult for the family and us.

Anne was also successful in her career. For more than 25 years, she ran a division of Medicare for the government. She jokes that when she retired they created a new department of 30 people to replace her. She is articulate and confident. She is also disarmingly honest in sharing the ups and downs of her days trying to manage his steady decline. The hardest part of this has been a change in personality. She states that before the onset of dementia, Clint was a kind, gentle man. He was an attentive husband and father. She adds, "He now is impulsive, angry and maddeningly oppositional."

They lost a grandson to a freak infection after a bone marrow transplant for sickle cell. The pain from this has been unbearable. The entire family suffers from PTSD from this sudden loss. Clint has been hit the hardest. He is obsessed with the grandson's death and speaks of it several times a day, often tearfully.

We have been caring for him for nearly 2 years. They return for a 3-month followup. When I enter, she greets me with a smile. We are friends now and the formality of a typical doctor's appointment are long gone. We share a bond, an affection for her husband and an uneasiness with where this is headed.

CHE: How are we doing?

AWD: We are slipping. Lots of stuff to talk about.

CHE: Give me the positives first.

AWD: Several positives. I see the medication working. He is less anxious and he may be less obsessed with money and people stealing it. He also loves the day care center where he goes, which is a godsend to me. I have 6 hours, 3 days a week to recharge.

CHE: When you say "slipping," what do you mean?

AWD: He is less aware, extremely quiet except to argue. I am losing him. He refuses to shower and will wear the same clothes for days at a time, even to bed. The obsession with our grandson is more intense and more frequent. Confusion is a problem every day.

CHE: How are you doing with all this? If the best day in your life was a 1, and not being able to take this any more and you are getting ready to jump off the Bank of America building is a 10, where are you?

AWD: It varies. Some days I am a 4, others I am an 8.

CHE: We always come back to four things to let us know how we are doing. You already know what I am going to say.

AWD: Calm, safe, clean and loved. He is not calm. Safety issues—driving, medications, wandering and scams. He is not clean. He is loved but it is getting hard. The man that loved me is gone. I love him but it is hard to remember those times that worked. Every day is a checklist.

I want you to know what has happened to me. I had my 75th birthday this past week. I woke up that morning with this strange feeling. I realized that something had to give. I am caring for my 94-year-old mother. My husband, who is declining in front of my eyes, needs more vigilance. And my daughter is getting a divorce and needs more of me. I try to help her with the grandchildren as much as I can.

I realized that I would have to change, protect myself, in order to live up to all the demands being made of me. I had the feeling that I was nothing more than a reflection of the needs of those around me. I FELT I WAS DISAPPEARING. If I don't push back in some way, these demands will crush me. They may have already crushed me.

CHE: Wow. What did you do when you had this epiphany?

AWD: This new me was tested in exactly 10 minutes. My daughter called and asked if I could keep her daughters for the weekend. She had a chance to get away and desperately wanted to go. The new me said "No." The old me never said no. I surprised myself with this newfound resolve. I then did something totally out of character for me. I went online and ordered a pair of large, red glasses. Really big, really red. For some reason, I have always wanted them but would never have paid that much for anything so nonessential.

CHE: Get them out, put them on.

She reached into her purse and reverentially removed them from the even redder case and put them on.

AWD: [She laughed.] What do you think?

CHE: They are perfect.

AWD: I know what you are thinking. The red glasses symbolize my new determination to not disappear. Maybe, maybe not. I do feel stronger when I have them on. The real point here is that if I don't find new strength, the demands from my mother, husband and daughter will overwhelm me. That I am sure of. If the world knows not to mess with me when I have the glasses on, then they will have done their job.

CHE: You have always had the strength. The red glasses are just a reminder.

Ω

CLINT CONTINUES TO SLOWLY decline. Driving becomes a major issue. He initially was restricted to driving during the day and only in familiar surroundings. The most recent testing revealed that he had dropped close to a level that would prevent him from driving. We needed a strategy. He was not going to make this easy. It would take all hands on deck to make him safer. I asked Anne who had the most leverage with Clint. She answered, "Without question, my daughter Lisa." We scheduled a family conference with Anne, Lisa and me.

My impression of Lisa was formed by one sentence in a meeting with her mother. She wanted to go away for the weekend and Anne had stood her ground. I probably had a faintly negative view of Lisa based on that random comment but knew that we needed her desperately to deal with her father.

I walk in to the conference room not knowing what to expect. Lisa is sitting across the table next to her mother. Her hair is pulled back in an "all business" manner. This features her pretty face, reminiscent of her mother's.

She smiled. "Mom has already told me she sold me out as the unappreciative daughter who is the bottom half of her caregiver sandwich."

Anne puts on the red glasses.

CHE: Lisa, you don't have a pair of the red glasses, do you?

LMD: No. I don't need them to make me more assertive. I have plenty of that already.

CHE: Tell me about yourself. [I learn that she has a degree from UNC-Chapel Hill and is a VP at one of the banks. She lost her son one year ago. She now is raising her two daughters, ages 11 and 13, alone.]

LMD: My marriage did not survive losing our son. My dad was an amazing father and we have lost him a little each day over the past year. We are all reeling from these tragic events. Happiness just seems to be postponed for everyone in our family. Watching dad decline and seeing his despondency is a persistent reminder of everything we have lost.

CHE: What do you see?

LMD: My mother is overwhelmed. She has risen to every demand made of her but there are limits to what wounded individuals can endure. She is effective and loving with her mother and with my daughters but she has trouble standing up to my dad. His confusion is dominating every day. He always knows me but there are times when he is not sure who his granddaughters are. The day care has helped but my major concern is his driving. I won't let my children ride with him and therefore he should not be on the road. The medications are marginally helping. I wonder if higher doses would help even more.

CHE: I agree with your take on this. We will address the driving. He is already scheduled to receive higher doses of the medications. We may need to add one more to combat the anger. I am impressed with both of you refusing to have these travails break you. Lisa, I want you to get a pair of the red glasses. They are a sign of extraordinary endurance which is rare in this world. You have earned them along with my full respect.

Ω

If there is a more powerful example of the oft-related "sandwich effect," I haven't seen it. Mother caring for mother, husband, daughter and granddaughters. Daughter caring for grandmother, mother, dad and daughters.

On a recent visit, I asked Lisa, "What keeps you going?"

She responded, "There is so much on all our plates that I just try to get through today. I don't think about tomorrow or when this nightmare will end. I just match my wits and strength with the demands of this day. One foot in front of the other. I have no other options. I am strong."

Strong indeed.

A Silver Star For Donna

I would give anything to start this story with the disclaimer you see in most modern books of fiction: *The characters in this story are not real, they are fictitious. Any resemblance to any living person is unintended.* But I cannot. This story is true. With permission, I have not changed any names or details.

It is 1966. Donna Ciccone has been discharged from the hospital at West Point after a week's stay for appendicitis. She is from a military family stationed close by. She is shopping in the Post Exchange before going home.

A cadet with a huge black eye comes up to her out of the blue and nervously utters a line that has never worked and will never work (except this once). "Haven't we met somewhere before?"

The answer is no. He explains that the shiner is from head trauma from rugby.

Donna just had her first encounter with Cadet Michael Norton. He proved to be an ardent and persistent pursuer from that day on.

This was not love at first sight. But letters are exchanged and Donna accepts an invitation to a football weekend. They date several times before he graduates in May 1967.

Michael arrived in Vietnam in December 1967 as a second lieutenant in the Artillery. He functioned as a forward observer, guiding artillery fire toward the enemy. He was often in close proximity to the enemy—and in close proximity to Agent Orange.

From March 3-7, 1968, Captain Norton was involved in action that would change him forever. Several times during that four-day period, he exposed himself to enemy fire to save a platoon of American soldiers trapped by the enemy. For these four days of daring and courage, Michael Norton was awarded the Silver Star, the third highest military decoration for valor in combat. He never mentioned it to anyone.

Michael went on to medical school at Wake Forest and he and Donna Ciccone were married. He completed a residency in anesthesiology. They had two children. He joined a practice in Charlotte, N.C., and remained there for 25 years. His partners to a person gave him high praise as a physician (caring and prepared) and a man (principled and fun). He had a storybook life. Until he didn't.

Donna chooses her words with care and caution, which makes her an unusually effective communicator with details and emotion. In our five years of chats, she is often crying and laughing at the same time, symbolizing coexisting pain and strength.

$$\Omega$$

DN: What has been so agonizing is the fact that all our dreams came true. We came so close to having it all and it just all fell apart, quickly. I'm not talking about the material stuff. I'm talking about the bond we had with each other. It went deep on love, respect, fun. We had this all planned out. And then… Looking back, there were subtle signs that something had changed. But at the time there was no alarm. Michael was always on the quiet side, always the stoic soldier.

CHE: What was the first thing you saw that gave you concern and when did it happen?

DN: It was more than five years ago. We were on our way to his class reunion at West Point, the highlight of every year. We always drove to Charlottesville, Va., the first night. We are creatures of habit. We stayed in the same hotel and always ate at the same restaurant. Michael dropped me off and went to park the car. After waiting 20 minutes at the table alone, I had this premonition that something terrible had happened. Not just that he had gotten turned around but a feeling of foreboding for him and our future. This was the first time I felt the dread that accompanied every search to find him. I had no idea that this was about to become my life, constant searches, constant dread.

I found him that night. But I never really got an explanation of what happened. For a long time, I thought he might have fallen again and this was all from another concussion.

Things began to unravel. One morning he awoke and did not know who I was. He could not be convinced that I was his wife, Donna. He thought I was another Donna.

Ω

This was our first encounter. I enter the room. The two people I confront are well known to me. Dr. Norton was an anesthesiologist. In my former role as a cardiac surgeon, he put my patients to sleep countless times over the past 25 years.

He was always prepared and stayed calm in tense situations. I always felt good about having him with me, especially in high-risk situations.

I had not seen him since he had retired. He greets me with a smile and look of recognition. It is not clear that he grasps why he is here or why I have come into the room.

Donna immediately reacts to the fact that they are here to see me because of some sort of dementia. She tears up. Her voice cracks. She quickly recovers and greets me with a strong voice and dry eyes.

CHE: Colonel, how are you doing? Is retirement what you expected? Lots of time at the beach?

Michael: I'm not sure what you mean. I guess I'm doing OK.

I ask a few more questions and try to hit on a subject that clicks. No luck. There is no spontaneous speech, no appropriate response.

Michael leaves with my nurse, Shelly, to be tested. I am alone with Donna. Her tears reappear.

DN: He doesn't even know who I am. He calls me Donna, but the 48 years of our marriage are gone. This man who has been almost obsessed with me for most of his life thinks I am someone who works where he lives. I am Donna, but not THE Donna. It is too much. The pain is excruciating. What is this? Have you seen it before?

CHE: Yes, Donna, this is a delusion. It is called the Capgras delusion. We have several patients with it. It is described as the patient thinking that their spouse or a person close to them has been replaced by an imposter. They look identical but one is a fake. It can come and go. A delusion is a false, fixed belief. The key word is fixed. You cannot reason him out of the delusion.

DN: Believe me, I have tried. If anger could fix this, we would be over it. I have tried everything. What caused this?

CHE: We are not always certain. In our practice, we have seen it as the result of a stroke. Some of our patients with it have had serial concussions. It can be associated with vascular dementia. Michael has two major risk factors for dementia—the concussions and his exposure to Agent Orange.

DN: Do you see a lot of Vietnam veterans with dementia? Do they have exposure to Agent Orange? [1,2]

CHE: Yes. They present with atypical symptoms but the progression is unrelenting. We also see the co-morbid conditions—Kaposi sarcoma, Parkinson's and associated malignancies. Michael is the first Vietnam veteran we have seen with Capgras syndrome but we have many in different stages of dementia.

DN: Along with this he has another delusion. He will say, "I don't live here. I live in a place exactly like this but it is somewhere else." Have you seen that also?

CHE: Yes. It is called *reduplicative paramnesia.* It is a marker for wandering. If left alone, he will go.

DN: His "escaping" has become too much to handle. I have to search for him several times a week despite never leaving him alone. Strangely, he is still resourceful, even sly in his attempts to "get away." My life is now dominated by these delusions. I am the strange woman who finds him running away, begging him to get in the car before he gets run over. I can't sleep, fearing he has left the house. If the door opens, an alarm goes off but even that safety measure doesn't reassure me.

CHE: Do you think your setup at home is working? Is he safe?

DN: If you are asking me if I am ready to place him somewhere away from me, the answer is no. He would never give up on me and I am not giving up on him. Is it too much? Yes. Am I rational? No.

CHE: At this point, we have four obligations to him. We want him calm, safe, clean and loved. I think we are doing good on the love part. Does he resist showering and personal hygiene?

DN: Yes, in certain situations. You have to pick your times but he will shower if I insist. He is not sure why this stranger cares whether he bathes, but I am marginally successful on this one.

CHE: There are seven safety issues. The first two are non-negotiable. Driving and firearms.

DN: He no longer is driving, doesn't even ask to drive. There are no firearms in the house.

CHE: Then we have the stove, medications and falls.

DN: The stove is not a problem. I manage the medications. He is still athletic. Believe me, he can still run when he wants to.

CHE: Finally, we have wandering and scams.

DN: He tries to run away any chance he gets. It is my main concern every minute of the day. He is obsessed that he is running out of money. Often the "breakouts" are attempts to get to the bank. I go over finances several times a day to lower his anxiety. This has become less effective as he has worsened.

CHE: I know you are aware of why wandering is one of the major signs that he is not safe at home. You are also experiencing the exhaustive effect it has on anyone living in that home.

DN: I got it. Just not ready to fold. I have to be close to protect him. I am here to preserve even the few shreds of dignity we have left.

We separate and I go in to examine Michael, review his testing and talk with him. The exam is unremarkable. Heart, lungs and gross neuro exam are normal. He tests poorly on the neuro-cognitive test with a total score of 13/30. Deficiencies are short-term memory, executive function, abstraction and orientation (date, month, year, etc.) There are no signs of Parkinson's disease on his initial exam.

CHE: Michael, who is with you today?

MSN: Donna.

CHE: Who is Donna?

MSN: She is a person who works where I live.

CHE: Are you married to her?

MSN: No, she is not my wife Donna. I would know my own wife.

CHE: Where *is* your wife Donna?

MSN: She is away.

We cover several topics, including exposure to Agent Orange and the effect it can have on the brain. He recalls the exposure to Agent Orange and knows that he has had two major concussions but has no details of those injuries. I explain how those injuries can result in our brains playing tricks on us, specifically thinking that his wife is another Donna. The fixed part of the delusion dominates. He assures me that this woman is not his wife.

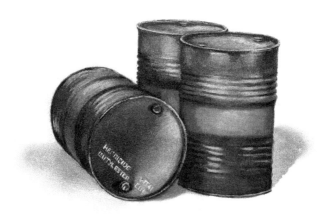

Ω

THIS INITIAL EVALUATION CAME more than five years ago. We started medication that had the potential to make the delusions less frequent and less intense. They worked marginally. As his confusion increased, so did his agitation and aggression. Medication to calm him helped but did not eliminate the constant urge to escape. His situational awareness declined dramatically. He became quiet, offering no spontaneous speech. Early on, remnants of his once gentle, kind and fun-loving personality survived, just enough to remind Donna of who he was, what he had accomplished. These quickly disappeared.

I see him every three months. Slowly, Parkinsonian features begin to creep into my exams. Parkinson's disease is a common indication of poisoning from Agent Orange. His voice became soft. He rarely blinked. His movements slowed. A once athletic gait became a shuffle. His arms were motionless at his sides. His arms and legs resisted movement, exhibiting increasing rigidity.

It is common in caring for patients declining at such a rapid pace that the principal caregiver suffers a change in empathy. A switch is thrown. They don't throw it—it is thrown *for* them.

They step off the emotional roller coaster. Compassion is separated from commitment. The checklist of things to do is still intact and all the boxes checked. But the heart-wrenching torment of watching up close someone you love suffer is now from a distance. Humans can only take so much of the raw sensitivity present early in such a tragedy. The distance allows the caregiver to breathe and to execute the care. Without it, sustaining the level of care required—which only increases—becomes harder.

For Donna, there would be no distance—she never experienced the change in empathy. The tragedy evokes raw emotion, anger and helplessness every second of every day.

She kept him at home for 3½ of these five years. He was never sure of who she was and why she was there. Finally, the anger, confusion, exit-seeking and exhaustion won. She spent a year looking at every memory care facility within 20 miles. A VA facility would provide Army buddies but it was too far away.

I wish I could say that we found the perfect place, but I can't. The disease is progressing and he is more difficult to manage. Remember, he is a warrior. We have been in the emergency room countless times for agitation and aggression. While at the ER, we are informed that the facility where he lives is refusing to take him back. A frantic search for a safe haven, for professionals who can handle a patient exhibiting Michael's symptoms, was always an unrealized expectation. It has been torture.

The irony of it all is that at times, Donna is more vulnerable and fragile. Two minutes later, she is stronger and even more formidable. She will fight this to the end. We have a text trail that reflects all this emotion and resolve. The text trail is also evidence that she has not lost her sense of humor. I have to remind her that oppositional defiance on her part is not an effective caregiver strategy.

We are now close to the end. Michael is bedridden and can no longer communicate with anyone. Thankfully, he sleeps 20 hours a day. I will be relieved to finally get the call that his suffering is over. There will be a life for Donna after this ordeal. She and I both know that it will take time to develop. She is aware that loving Michael, fighting his illness and refusing to give in to his decline has changed her forever. Life has nothing harder to throw at her.

The throes of his illness—the ups, downs, countless hours in the ER, getting kicked out of facilities for his aggression, watching him decline—have been too much. Donna knew that from the beginning. Now when I think of her, I see her alone, afraid and defiant. This ordeal has stripped away everything but the vital elements but among these sinews is irrepressible resolve and courage.

What comes to mind is Michael exposing himself to enemy fire over those four days long ago in Vietnam. Same thing on Donna's part—but it's been far longer than four days. In the military, we recognize such valor with medals, symbols of honor and respect. For the rest of us, we just have to know it when we see it.

Go ahead, Donna. Put it on. You earned that Silver Star.

Ω

Michael Norton passed away on April 21, 2023. He is buried at the U.S. Military Academy at West Point, N.Y., surrounded by his fellow fallen cadets.

Donna is cautiously regaining her balance. She has no capacity for deceit and, when asked, will admit that at this early point she is not sure where her life is heading.

"On some days, I have never felt stronger," she says. "On other days, never more unsure."

She will figure this out. She always has. What she does know is that life will never be what it was and she will never be who she was. The demands and pain of the past seven years have set a new life into motion—a new life emboldened by two powerful takeaways.

First, having survived this tragic sequence, her fear is gone. She will survive on her terms. What this will look like we are not yet sure. Second, the experience, the suffering, has opened avenues of emotion and connections to other humans. These new links are the building blocks for what is to come in her new life.

Summary

The first five chapters are included in Part 1, Background. Each chapter serves an important role in setting up what follows.

We opened on the riverbank with a Bedouin tribe trying to survive. The takeaway was realizing that every tribe, including ours, deals with the same demands. They might have different answers but the questions are the same.

By focusing on the stark realities they face and the annual proximity to death, my intent is to foster a deeper understanding of the decisions we make and their consequences in similar straits.

Raymond Carver shared his final thoughts and assured us that affirmation from other humans is crucial at the end. We learned what defines the stage of life that, after his poem, I call the *late fragment*, who's in it and why.

I have included caregivers with the caveat that they may not qualify. But by assuming the care of an individual in the late stage of life, their lives are placed on an unwanted hold. The emotional toll cannot be minimized. Close to 20% of caregivers in our clinic die *before the identified patient*. This is a testament to the often devastating impact of watching this up close.

We now enter Part 2, Jeopardy. In Chapters 6–10, we confront the challenges inherent in late aging. Each aging individual, if they live long enough, will face some or all of them. There is no "get-out-of-jail-free card" here. How one responds to these certain snags will determine a person's late-in-life relevance, happiness and connectivity to other humans.

I have spent close to three years living in the *Late Fragment*. I have been there with individuals from my past. I have been there with my patients and their families. I have been there with aging individuals who allowed me to interview them, then allowed me to be their confidant, and finally their friend.

The honesty and candor of these sages has revealed to me the fundamentals of aging. What are the questions each of us need to ask before we leave this world? What do we do with the answers to those questions?

Before we get into the answers, we need to know the liabilities, traps and obstacles that await us, often lurking. What do these barriers look like? When are they likely to appear? If we are unaware about the presence of dangers, naïve to being in jeopardy, our efforts to avoid them will be either inadequate or late.

Part II
Jeopardy

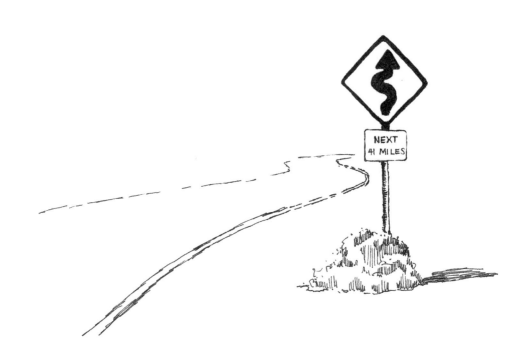

6

The Sin of Pride

Sorrow makes children of us all.

Ralph Waldo Emerson

This chapter is a cautionary tale. It contains many of the predictable elements that long lives are forced to confront, and the consequences when the response to those elements go awry.

First, let me introduce Randal Myers Ranson (RMR). He is an 82-year-old retired lawyer who makes an appointment in our clinic. When asked his reason for wanting to be seen, he answers, "I have concerns over memory and life in general."

Randal practiced law until age 77 when he quit to care for his wife, Audrey, who was diagnosed with pancreatic cancer. She was dead within one year of the diagnosis. He was married to her for 56 years, 55 of them perfect, he says. He was raised by a religious family on a tobacco farm in eastern North Carolina. He left home at 17 to attend Davidson College. He was the first person in his family to graduate from high school let alone attend college. After graduation from Davidson, he entered Duke Law School. He was an honors student at both institutions. He was recruited by a prestigious Charlotte law firm and stayed there 55 years. All the boxes are checked: Athletics, military service, career, community service and church. He was a respected lawyer and is still revered in diverse circles throughout Charlotte. I know from the data collected following his first visit that his neuropsychological testing is above average for his age. The brain MRI was normal. So were his labs.

He is nervous upon entering. He is dressed casually but with concern for the details of dress. He speaks softly and chooses his words carefully. He makes consistent eye contact. His language is fluid and effective. Initially, there were no smiles. He begins a monologue with the words and sentences coming fast, as if there is a time limit on how long he has to speak.

RMR: I am actually embarrassed to be here. I know there are people in real need and my troubles should not be anyone's concern. But I have to say, I have lost my way and I am hoping you can help me. Up until my wife left (interesting word choice), I thought I was doing OK. This is the fourth year I have been without her and things are not getting better. I am burdened with this profound fatigue that I cannot shake. I feel sad all the time. I seem to be nervous all the time. I walk around the house looking for something but I have no idea what I am looking for or even why I would need it. Everything seems out of focus. I either can't do things or don't want to do things. I'm not sure which.

CHE: Tell me, where are you living?

RMR: I live alone in the house I have lived in for nearly fifty years. It's where we raised our daughter. Up until now, I have been happy there.

CHE: Is your weight stable?

RMR: No, it's down. I weigh 132. I used to stay around 150.

CHE: Tell me about your diet.

RMR: I try to get one full, healthy meal per day. I go to Publix but come home with less than ideal choices. My ability to plan and execute is bad. I eat a lot of snack food, peanuts etc. I get food to take home. It just doesn't seem to last long enough.

CHE: How much alcohol are you drinking?

RMR: Very little. I have never been a drinker.

CHE: On any given day when you say "This is going to be a good day because I get to do this," what would this be?

RMR: To be honest, I have lost interest in almost everything. I loved golf. When my wife was alive, we had a busy social life. There was always something going on, dinners, plays, weekends away with friends. It is all gone. Nothing seems to matter.

CHE: How do you sleep?

RMR: Fitfully. I will awaken at 2 a.m. with my mind filled with dread. I am forced to get up and I walk around the house. Sad things, memories of bad times, are front and center in my brain. When I wake up in the morning, I am exhausted. Sleep doesn't touch my fatigue.

CHE: How many days a week do you go without contact with another human being?

RMR: Does waving at the lady next door count?

CHE: No.

RMR: Often four, sometimes five.

CHE: Do you have any regrets about the care you gave your wife during her illness?

RMR: No. When I saw her suffering and in pain, I wanted it to stop. I probably wasn't perfect but I stopped everything to attend to her. No, I have no regrets over that period of my life. The illness dominated everything. Every day there was either a mini crisis or a major crisis which kept all in turmoil. My regrets came after she was gone.

It was only after she was gone that misgivings gathered to make me sad. I realized she was the center of everything of value in our lives. I was under the false impression that my career and the troubles of others were as important if not more important than the simple things that occurred at home. She teed up life for me. I got to see, react, appreciate and be involved because of her. She was the action. I was a passive follower. She loved me enough to allow me to live that illusion without one shred of jealousy or animosity. She was gone and I was left with regret that I didn't see it when she was alive. I could have, should have, done better. She should have felt special. Who do I offer this apology to? Where do I go to get away from this torment? I am stuck and terribly sad.

I am guilty of the sin of pride. I thought that what I was doing for others was so important. I took immense pride in the success of my career and the respect it brought. I should have done better. She was amazing and I fear she left this world without her knowing how amazing she was. It's too late now.

CHE: Have you thought about hurting yourself? Not wanting to be here? Living with this pain must be hard.

RMR: I want to say no. But I can't. I have asked God to take me. I see no reason to continue this. I have no hope the future will be different.

CHE: Have you thought about how you would do this?

RMR: Again, I want to say no. But I can't. There's a leftover prescription from my wife's illness. It would be a simple instrument. It's in the medicine chest. I feel weak, diminished. I come from proud, strong people. My father would be ashamed of me. I have lost contact with myself. The pride I took from my roles in life is gone. That person, for all practical purposes, has disappeared.

CHE: Tell me about family.

RMR: I have a daughter in Houston, Texas. She has one daughter who is going off to University of Texas. COVID 19 has isolated me from them. For two years, our involvement has been over the phone. They have busy lives and I refuse to dump my problems on them.

CHE: Have you been honest with them about your recent struggles?

RMR: No.

Ω

I WANTED YOU TO meet Randal for several reasons. First, he is an example that no one, not even the most successful among us, are immune to the travails of life. One day, things are in order, predictable, happy. One sentence from a doctor and the entire structure comes crashing down. Randal's story and the eventual outcome hopefully can serve as an example for the potential of healing and replacing despair with hope.

Second, he personifies many of the pitfalls and downsides of late aging. We are going to discuss each of these in detail. Knowing there are land mines and where they are is key to avoiding them and moving beyond them.

But first, how do we help him? The approach at Memory & Movement Charlotte would involve three steps.

The first: Immediate.

CHE: First, let me assure you. You do not have dementia. But we are in trouble as you have already admitted and acted on by being here. This regret, what you call "the sin of pride,"[1] is no longer rational. It has become an obsession, a destructive force. It will take time to regain our balance. I will need total buy-in, meaning that you say, "I want help and will do what you say."

RMR: I am in. Tell me what I need to do.

CHE: The first thing is go home and bring me the narcotic pills. Drive straight back and hand them to me. Are there any firearms in the house?

RMR: No.

CHE: Tomorrow morning at 9 a.m. a lady will ring your doorbell. Her name is Joclyn Kendig. She is a case manager who works with us. She will interview you, assess the situation and make recommendations. She will arrange for a caregiver to come four mornings a week for four hours. This lady will clean, shop with you, prepare meals and escort you anywhere you want to go. She is there to ensure that you are up, healthy and have access to everything you need, especially food. Lastly, I will need permission to speak with your daughter in Texas.

I am going to start you on a medication, Lexapro. The goal will be to decrease the anxiety and agitation that is keeping you stirred up. It will also break the obsessions that are dominating your mind all day, every day. It also may help with sleep as the anxiety and obsessions calm down. We will start low. But if you tolerate it, we will steadily move you to a higher dose. We will have to get closer until I feel you are stronger. The first counseling session is the first of next week. I need you to promise me two things: First, any downturn with negative thoughts or plans to hurt yourself will trigger a call to me. Second, I want you to attend church this Sunday. Am I right that you have been a member of a church and served in leadership in the past?

RMR: Yes. What do I say when people ask me, "Where have you been?"

CHE: Just say, "I have had some recent health problems but it feels good to be back here." I have great hopes for your future. But the return from this despair is not going to depend on medication or my advice. The future for you depends on your controlling the conversation that you have with yourself. It will demand that you actively filter out negativity and discover reasons why you want to live and what you want that life to look like. We are going to take some baby steps. Nothing earth-shattering. Yet!

The counseling sessions occurred over several months. I am condensing them to highlight the important points.

Five days later...

CHE: Did you make it to church?

RMR: Yes, I did. I only went to the service and sat in back. I was nervous the whole time. I felt out of place.

CHE: Did you see any of your old friends?

RMR: Yes. Several people got up to greet me when I slipped in. My thoughts the entire time, "I may look like your old friend but I am an imposter." I was gratified by two old friends wanting to get together. I was reluctant to commit to anything.

I know why you wanted me to go. I told you that I had lost touch with myself. I had forgotten who I was. You were hoping that when I saw familiar people it would start the process of remembering me to me. Not yet.

CHE: Baby steps. Nothing forced.

RMR: Lots of activity at my house. Joclyn showed up, then the caregiver Roz. They emptied my refrigerator and both took me to the grocery store. I have enough prepared meals for a week. They parted all the curtains, opened the windows. And I must say it felt good to see the sunshine and have fresh air in the house. It was a sign I had become a recluse. They are pros. They treated me with a soft touch. I thought they would make me feel helpless, a troubled old man. I hate to admit it, but I am looking forward to their next visit.

CHE: I had a long talk with your daughter, Sophie. You apparently are good at faking. She has been concerned about your isolation but was not aware of how dire things have gotten. I am sure she called you.

RMR: You sold me out. She was not happy with me. COVID 19 has prevented me from seeing both Sophie and my granddaughter, Natalie, for nearly two years. It is apparent that the interval was a bigger deal than I realized. We are making plans. But, just saying, I am not going to be a burden to my family under any circumstances.

CHE: The burden came from my call to your daughter and the shock that you had not been honest with her. I also got to know your wife, Audrey, through Sophie. It has given me needed insight into you and your marriage.

RMR: Great. Just what I need, an exposé on my life. What's next, an article in *People* magazine?

CHE: Just a touch of sarcasm and the last vestiges of a sense of humor. We are making progress. First, bring me up to date. How are you dealing with these intrusions? Are we making matters worse?

RMR: Do you want me to say that I am ecstatic with all the attention, even though I know it is well-intentioned? I feel shame that I have gotten to this point and lost control. You said that any hope of recovery depends on my thoughts and, I think you said, the conversation I have with myself. Trying to see life with positive spin. I am nowhere near that. We still haven't gotten to the real problem. What exactly has gotten me into this mess? I know dozens of men who have lost their wives. They all seem to struggle for a while, but then rally. It has been three years since Audrey left and I have gotten worse. I'm thinking I'm out of bullets. Sorry, bad choice of words in my predicament. Sorry.

CHE: OK, let's get to it. As you said, sadly people go through the loss of loved ones every day. Why can't you get your balance back? What is different about this loss compared to others?

First, let me define this. Medically, we call this an abnormal grief reaction. In your case, the reaction to Audrey's death has been longer, deeper and more intense than would have been predicted. Abnormal grief reactions are characterized by the loss triggering anxiety, depression and profound sadness that doesn't abate. It robs the survivor of any satisfaction with the life that is left and robs them of hope for the future. It also tragically steals the pleasure from memories of past. The loss and details surrounding it become an obsession that dominates all thought and action.

Each situation is unique. You state clearly that you have no regrets over your care of Audrey during her illness. You also share that 55 years of your 56-year marriage were perfect, the last being brutal with her decline.

RMR: She was amazing in all aspects especially as a mother and a wife. She was also grandmother of the century.

CHE: Your regrets center on your realizing after her death how central she was to everything important in your lives. From Sophie's description, she did things effortlessly and unselfishly, with joy. I can see how you would miss her dreadfully. You said, "I missed it. I should have seen all this when she was alive and made her feel special."

RMR: She should have known how I loved her and felt it before she died. I think of all the times I thought things that she would have loved to hear from me and I never said them. I feel the sin of pride. Thinking too much about career and being proud of being accomplished and not even being aware of the simple things that mattered so much.

CHE: I can understand how you would punish yourself over not seeing her vital role. You have high expectations from every aspect of your life. Careers demand time and attention, often to the detriment of more worthy pursuits. I am not going to try to dissuade you from these feelings. What I am going to do is point out that these regrets are misgivings you have about yourself. "I could have done better" is the mantra. Let's take a look at Audrey and get her perspective.

I never met her. I only know her through you and your daughter, Sophie. I know speaking of her and about her are almost sacred at this point. I assure you I am choosing my words carefully and respectfully.

RMR: Thank you.

CHE: If you will humor me for just a few minutes, I would like to do a short role play. Since Audrey's thoughts and feelings are central to the regret you feel, I think we need to get her take on your predicament. We need to ask Audrey a few questions.

I have asked your daughter the same questions. The content and tone of my responses will reflect Sophie's thoughts and opinions as well as yours. If I am off, stop me.

First question: Audrey, did you feel loved and respected within your family? Daughter Sophie would say, "Absolutely."

Second question: Were you aware that on occasion your husband had difficulty expressing his true feelings? Did the distraction of his law practice and his desire to be successful in his career ever compete with your family agenda? My answer comes from Sophie and the insight I have gleaned from our visits.

Audrey's "Answer": *Absolutely not. My husband is the son of a tobacco farmer from Sampson County, N.C. He has been on his own since he left home at 17. The life he was entering was foreign to everyone and everything that had gone before him. He was and is on his own. He keeps his own counsel. I knew he needed me on many fronts. I loved completing him. I knew when he looked at me and approved of me and the life we had together that he was in touch with his emotions. They just weren't connected to his tongue. His life was a quest to prove himself worthy of the respect of his peers. He was driven to succeed. I filled in the rest. We were a great team.*

RMR: Doc, you are killing me here. It is almost like she is here with us.

CHE: Here is where this is going to get tough. When you and I first spoke, I came away with one goal. That goal was to open your eyes and show you the reasons you have to live.

The third and last question: Audrey, what gave your life purpose? If you were able on your way out to turn to your husband and offer one final heads up, what would you say?

Audrey's "Answer": We have had a great life. It produced a daughter and granddaughter who are symbols of our devotion to each other and the time we had together. Take care of them.

CHE: Randal, I know you know where I am going with this. I have probably overstepped my clinical bounds with the conversation we just had. I don't have to connect all the dots. I do want to connect two. First, turn toward the living—your daughter, granddaughter and everyone else important in your life. When I say turn toward the living, I include you. Every person who has ever lost a spouse has regrets. No one is perfect. The happier the marriage, the closer the couple, the more regret.

The second connecting of the dots. The day you brought those pills back to the office and handed them to me, you didn't really hand them to me. You handed them to *Audrey*.

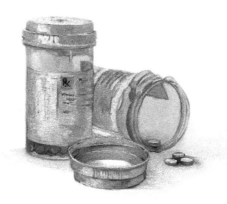

Six months later:

CHE: Tell me how things are going?

RMR: You already know I am doing better. I am sleeping well. My weight is back to normal. It is still a struggle to connect socially with friends. I have pushed myself, at your insistence, but it is awkward. This is where I really miss Audrey. She always made me look good when I was anxious. What has made the most difference is seeing my daughter and granddaughter. I talk to my daughter several times a week. Both have visited. I am still lonely but less so.

CHE: Would you say that overall the anxiety is down? Are there more positive thoughts?

RMR: Certainly fewer negative thoughts. I am better overall.

CHE: Those thoughts of "not wanting to be here," are they gone?

RMR: No, but definitely less intense and less frequent.

CHE: How many days a week are you alone? Having caregivers coming in doesn't count.

RMR: This has been my biggest challenge. I have never been a social starter. I would say three or four. I am enjoying nine holes of golf and lunch with old friends.

CHE: Now that you are alone, have you thought about going into a retirement center?

RMR: I do not want to leave my house. I am comfortable there. My whole life is there. Most of the friends that Audrey and I had are in a facility now. They seem to be happy or should I say content. It is just not for me.

CHE: When you say your whole life is there, what do you mean?

RMR: I mean the memories of my family and the life we shared. Also all the stuff we accumulated. It is here in one place. I don't think I could part with it.

CHE: You have admitted to still being lonely. Is it unrealistic to think that a different situation may make that better?

RMR: I would be just as lonely in a retirement center. I don't want to move. Where would Sophie and Natalie stay when they visit?

CHE: Loneliness is a destructive sensation. It has short- and long-term consequences that can be devastating. I am going to plant a seed today. I think we need to be around more people and not as isolated. I am going to call Sophie and recruit her as an ally for a possible move. Sitting in your house surrounded by stuff is not a life.

One year later

Randal is still at home. But a recent softening of resistance indicates that we may finally be gaining ground. The family involvement has been a game-changer.

I know after meeting this nice, sensitive man, you think this chapter is mis-titled. Randal was out to prove himself worthy of the respect and responsibilities that the world showered on him. His torment is not because of pride in his accomplishments. At least, not the sin he *thinks* he has committed. He had a great marriage and a successful career. The legacy, even with his wife's sudden illness, should not be catastrophic regret. How did we get here?

The perfect storm of her rapid exit and the social isolation from COVID 19 resulted in his profound loneliness. The absence of human contact prevented his being supported emotionally and reassured that he was a loving and valued husband. If he had been able to see Sophie and Natalie and felt their love and shared their loss, this whole affair would have been avoided. Negative thoughts manifested as regret became an unopposed obsession. Human interaction was the antidote.

Randal *did* have the sin of pride. But he is off on the source.

His being too proud to ask for help early as his life slipped away was the root of that sin.

Emerson was prescient when he wrote "Sorrow makes children of us all." Randal knew what Emerson meant because he lived it. The value system he used to judge himself didn't come from his stellar education or his distinguished career. Those triumphant intervals provided no solutions or guidance. When he lost touch with himself, those phases waned and his role in them disappeared. What came forth were the lessons from that long-ago abandoned life as a child from a religious family on a tobacco farm in eastern North Carolina. There, pride is still a sin.

There is science behind all this. Let's take a look.

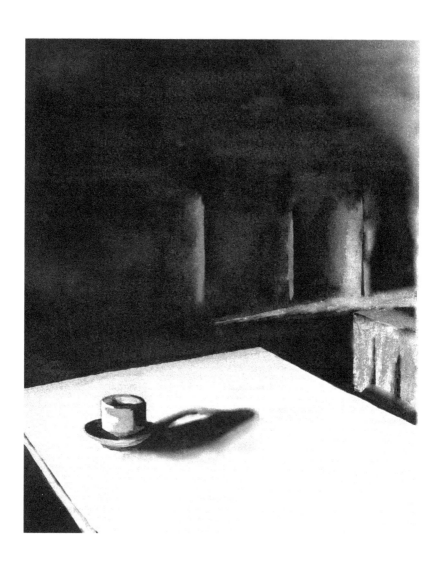

7

The Science of Despair

Human beings can withstand a week without
water, two weeks without food, many years of
homelessness, but not loneliness. It is the worst
of all tortures, the worst of all sufferings.

Paulo Coelho

One might assume that Randal's story would be rare. He presented with despondency and depression following the death of his wife. He had a prolonged, abnormal grief reaction complicated by personal regrets in his relationship with his wife. A strong, successful individual had lost touch with his former self and his family. The social isolation led to his feeling profoundly lonesome and abandoned. The depth of his torment was revealed in the statement, "The person I was is gone." He thought about suicide and how he would do it.

Is this an outlier?

It is not. The dramatic and surprising psychological challenges that besieged Randal after his wife's death are common, in fact more common than reported in the literature. Loneliness, depression and hopelessness overwhelmed an individual who was esteemed for his balance and insight. The unraveling of Randal is evidence of the power of these sinister forces. Let's take a look at the circumstances that allow these elements access to individuals and consider the warning signs when they are in play.

Living Alone[1-5]*

The cascade that devastated Randal began with the simple fact that he was living alone. According to the 2020 U.S. Census, 32% of individuals over 65 live alone. The number of aging individuals living alone has never been higher and is increasing throughout the world.

Living alone is the end point of multiple variables. It depends on your sex, your location in the world, whether you have lost a spouse for whatever reason, and obviously your age. Women are more likely to be alone because they often outlive their husbands. Single men are more likely to remarry. For women, the numbers are striking. At age 65, 21% of men live alone while 34% of women manage a solo household. Reaching the age of 75 increases the gap with 44% of women being alone.

An ideal situation for those in advancing age is the nearness of a multigenerational family. This is the norm in many regions of the world. Only 5% of Asian-Pacific, Middle Eastern and Sub-Saharan African adults live alone. In Western cultures, specifically Europe and the United States, 27% of those same aging adults live alone.

This does not mean that North American children care

---

* Endnotes in this chapter refer to multiple articles relating to the section topic.

less about their parents. It represents cultural responses to economic pressures that force individuals to leave home and often live significant distances from immediate family. This increases the probability of a parent living alone later in life.

In Randal's case, COVID 19 played a major role. The quarantine came late in his self-imposed exile but the timing and impact were devastating.

Randal was right when he blamed the sin of pride for his predicament. But he had its origin misplaced. He was too proud to admit to his daughter or anyone else that he was struggling. One can envision a better outcome if there had been better communication and contact with family or close friends. Being honest about his regrets and being able to TELL someone and then LISTEN to their take on it had the potential to limit the depths of the despondency.

We all at some level are defined by the interaction and opinions of other humans. An interaction with a valued friend had the potential to restore Randal's sense of himself and his lost value system. Sadly, the isolation prevented such a meeting.

Randal living alone resulted in the second step down in his decline—profound loneliness. A question that children with parents managing lives on their own should ask is, "Does the fact that I have a parent living alone necessarily mean they are lonely and not capable of managing that life effectively?"

The answer is NO. But it does increase the likelihood of loneliness being present. A follow-up is, "How will I know?" The answers lie in defining and understanding loneliness and its impact.

Loneliness[6-9]

First, we must distinguish loneliness from social isolation and solitude. Social isolation is the state of having minimal social contact with other humans. Solitude has the connotation of the isolation being voluntary and desired. Loneliness on the other hand is an emotional state reflecting the lack of desired interaction, closeness and affection of other humans. The key word is desired. The lonely person says. "I feel alone, isolated and diminished by being alone." But consider: I can be alone and not lonesome. I can also be lonesome in the constant company of friends and family.

Why is feeling lonely such a big deal? Don't all old people feel somewhat lonely?

No. Remember, we have defined loneliness as an emotional state which indicates a lack of desired affection and involvement with others. What are the red flags that would increase the likelihood of a parent feeling lonely?

The risk increases with the following factors—age alone, being female, widowed, divorced or alone for whatever reason. Declining mobility or an injury or illness of any kind can unravel a formerly acceptable domestic situation.

A pattern of isolation from family and friends signals decline. The number of days the person living alone goes without interacting with other humans is a barometer for the degree of isolation. One, maybe two days a week is acceptable. More than that is a major red flag.

The clues are often subtle. These would include making excuses for not sharing vacations or not visiting regularly. It may be a subtle change in the relationship with children or grandchildren. Repetitive questions and rapid forgetting may indicate cognitive decline.

Loneliness results in being less effective in managing a household, dramatic decreases in physical activity, loss of confidence and well-being. It is also directly related to depression, impaired cognition and the development of dementia.

Loneliness has measurable biological implications. The pathological isolation results in elevations in blood pressure, the core factor in cardiovascular health. Hypertension is the root cause of stroke, congestive heart failure, heart attacks and vascular dementia.

Suffering with unwanted social isolation is associated with obesity, diminished immunity and premature mortality. These vulnerabilities became evident when the coronavirus devastated this group worldwide.

Age alone is a chronic disease. It will take its toll. Individuals in their late 80s and early 90s face physical and cognitive decline that threaten their safety when living alone. One fall with injury can turn an almost ideal situation to unacceptable in an instant. Declining mobility both socially and physically indicate the need for continual vigilance and visits.

When loneliness is suspected in a parent or loved one, it is time to reevaluate and often intervene. The solution may be as simple as increasing visits by family members and involved friends. Predictable and certain interfaces and weekly dinners or outings make it more likely that the event will take place. More importantly, it allows the isolated individual to anticipate and rely on the attention. Other solutions may be more drastic, a move closer to family or entering a retirement facility to ensure more human contact.

In the case of Randal, the aftermath of unmitigated, unwanted isolation was major depression.

Depression[10-14]

Depression is a mood disorder that causes a persistent feeling of sadness and loss of interest in the details of life. It affects how you feel, think and behave. It eliminates hope for the future and robs one of the good and sustaining memories of the past.

Depression in the elderly is a major problem and grossly under-diagnosed. There are multiple levels of severity with depression. These range from situational depression, when mood and perspective are altered, to major depression, when symptoms interfere with work, sleep and decision-making.

When coupled with anxiety, which it often is, the impact on individual lives is compounded.

We are going to limit our discussion to major depression. The National Institutes of Health reported that 4.7% of individuals over age 50 were diagnosed with major depression in 2021. This represents more than five million people. One would assume that the incidence of major depression would continue to increase with advancing age given the many challenges of living long lives. While on the surface it might seem unlikely, only two million of those five million people were over age 65. One theory as to why is that major depression is linked to shorter lives. The survival data may reflect the attrition of lives from ages 50 to 65.

The incidence of major depression in those living alone is low. It is only when physical and cognitive decline are added that the numbers jump. Major depression accelerates the aging process, not only worsening the severity of the symptoms but undermining the capacity of the ailing individual to cope with the strain.

Women are more likely to be diagnosed with depression. This may reflect a willingness to admit to problems and seek help. It also stems from what we already know, that more women live alone, increasing the chance of loneliness.

The symptoms of depression are more nuanced in older individuals, making the diagnosis more difficult. It may involve a personality change characterized by irritability or anger. These alterations in mood and affect are often misattributed to age or the frustration of declining mobility. It misses the real culprit, clinical depression. Apathy and loss of pleasure from activities that previously gave great pleasure (anhedonia), are often present.

It is tragic that such a small percentage of depressed individuals seek help. Less than 3% of patients 65 and older receive treatment from a mental health professional. Primary care physicians recognize less than half of the significant depression in their patients.

This all leads to the fact that suicide in the elderly is linked to major depression. Each of the factors that led to the spiral downward that Randal suffered—living alone, loneliness and major depression—set the stage for his possibly taking his own life. Of these factors, the presence of depression and his refusal to seek help was the most powerful. Suicide in the elderly has its own profile. It is not rare.

Suicide[15-22]

It is not uncommon for older individuals to state, "I am ready to go. I have lived long enough." There is no cause for alarm in the majority of cases. In the clinical setting, however, further investigation is called for when a patient who is alone and has suffered the loss of a spouse states, "I don't know if I can keep going" or "I am ready for the Lord to take me." If when asked, "Have you thought about hurting yourself?" the choice of words and their intent become crucial to avoiding tragedy.

In our example with Randal, not only had he thought "about" hurting himself but "how" he would do it. Everything stops at this point. All options are in play, including emergency commitment if the threat is that dire. My instinct in his case was that Randal wanted to be stopped. That was why he was in front of me. The demand that he return with the pills was enough to end the immediate threat. It bought us time to work on solutions for the loneliness and depression that set this in motion.

The statistics regarding suicide in the elderly are well established but not widely known. Adults over the age of 65 make up 12% of the population but account for 17% of suicides. The scary numbers get scarier with advancing age. In a 2016 review, individuals ages 15 to 49 had an annual rate of suicide of 11.6 per 100,000 population. In the age group 50 to 69, the annual rate jumped to 16.7%. In those over 70, the rate was 27.45%.

What is more concerning is that these numbers grossly underestimate the true incidence of the problem. When an elderly person living alone is found dead in their home, the assumption is they died of natural causes. A heart attack or stroke is blamed. After all, they were elderly and that is what happens. In an alarming percentage of these discoveries, though, when no clues are provided as to why a person died, self-harm is involved. The numbers make the point: Suicide is common in the later stages of life, more common than reported.

Suicide not only has a different rate of occurrence in earlier stages in life, it has a different profile. A young person taking their life often is an impulsive act. Sinister chemicals produced by an event, insult or rejection flood the brain. This chemical reaction is tortuous and intolerable. In the mind of the individual, it must stop.

In the elderly, the process is planned, thought out often over an extended time period. No sudden impulsive act here. As a result, older adults are more successful in completing the intent. One in 4 suicide attempts in the elderly are completed compared with 1 in 200 in younger individuals.

At Memory & Movement Charlotte, we deal with the specter of suicide every day. In each patient, there is both an active and passive method used to assess the possibility of one harming themselves. The possibility of a suicide attempt is in the back of our minds. Often it is dismissed because of instinctive reassurances from the patient. I want to explain what propels concerns about self-harm to the front of our brains. The only reason to delve into this despair is to recognize the possibility of it occurring and preventing it. This sharing of what we do in the clinic is intended to alert and educate those who care for and care about these aging individuals who have gotten off track.

The evaluation begins before the patient arrives in the clinic. It begins with the phone call to make the appointment. Randal, when asked the purpose of his visit, said, "I am having problems with memory AND LIFE IN GENERAL." This was an unusual "chief complaint" that we note in the chart. I am alerted before I see him.

The initial impression that a patient makes on greeting staff and nurses is also noteworthy. The presence of a smile and animated speech calms most of our concerns.

When initial concerns are not calmed, the vigilance goes deeper. Direct questions are asked. "Have you ever thought about hurting yourself?" And the follow-up, "Have you thought about how?" Asking these questions is crucial. It allows the patient to "come clean" with their menacing thoughts and plans. It has been shown to be an effective preventive measure.

Now comes the hard part. By this time our concerns should be allayed in the majority of patients. If they are not, we have to assess the danger in front of us. Is the possibility this patient may hurt themselves real? Does it need immediate interventions? What are the factors that bear on our level of concern?

Our first concerns are emotional. Has there been a major loss of a loved one, spouse or a child? If present, is the grief reaction even remotely healthy and acceptable? Loss of loved ones, friends and family and our ability to endure those losses are the determinants of well-being as we age. This is a major theme in this book.

The second most important factor in determining risk of harm is physical decline and acute disabilities. Has the patient had a medical setback? Has this life changed irrevocably? The three factors that bear down on this are pain, mobility and fatigue. The possibility of a patient hurting themselves is directly related to their fear of the permanence of the situation.

The third major factor is financial. The impact of thinking "I am running out of money" cannot be overemphasized. It rivals the flood of chemicals that trigger sinister thoughts in younger individuals. There often is fear of "not having enough to eat."

Those of us caring for a patient with these forebodings often dismiss them, saying, "Don't be silly, surely we can reassure you that this won't happen." But fear undermines rational thought. These seemingly irrational thoughts are linked to the ubiquitous concerns over money that the aged seem to have. Take them seriously.

Certain demographics increase our vigilance. White males are more likely to consider suicide and choose violent exits. Individuals with a family history of a disease with progressive decline are at high risk for harm if they are diagnosed with that disease. We have to be especially strategic in the initial interchange with these people. Recent advances in the care related to the diagnosis need to be stressed with the patient.

In a clinic where we care exclusively for patients with memory challenges and Parkinson's disease, this situation comes up frequently.

Younger individuals still in mid-career who receive a diagnosis that will likely end that career are at extremely high risk for self-injury. If there is a family history of the disease, the risk rises. This requires close follow-up and often counseling sessions to ensure that balance and judgment prevail.

The legacy of suicide is a lifetime of pain and regret for all involved. It must be avoided. I hope that the takeaway from this discussion is being aware of the prevalence of suicide in those in the *late fragment*, and knowing the specific profiles that increase the need for vigilance.

The final element in dealing with the danger of suicide is having the tenacity to never let down the guards that can prevent these tragedies.

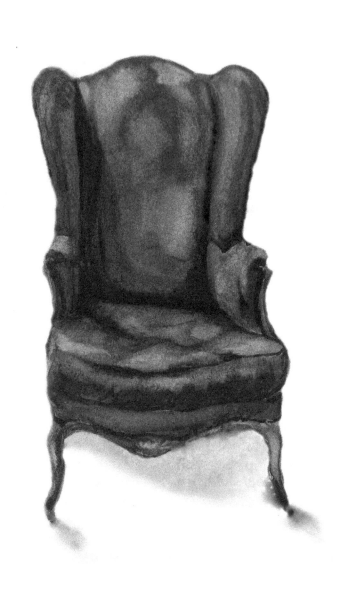

8

Beyond Sadness

Accepting losses and recovering from them is essential to surviving a long life. Each loss takes its toll in a different way. Consider the emotional devastation that follows the death of a life partner of fifty-plus years. The survivor's well-being and happiness is held in delicate balance until he or she decides what this new reality will look like. Understanding the factors in play is essential to an acceptable outcome.[1]

NTG is the widow of an orthopedic surgeon in Rock Hill, S.C. Her husband died seven years ago at age 62 from an unexpected cardiac event. He was diabetic and had a family history of cardiac disease. But the possibility that those two entities would team up to cause this tragedy never occurred to her. She had been with him since college. She took immense pride in her supporting role in his life and the starring role in the lives of her three children. The children, now in their 40s, all had successful careers and sadly lived in cities far from South Carolina.

It was always enough to be part of him, either at his side or waiting for him to return home. The children and grandchildren were precious to her, and she kept devoted friends from each stage of her life. But he was always the center of her multiple orbits. Even years after his death, she would tearfully and emphatically respond to the question "How are you doing?" by saying, "You don't understand. We breathed the same air."

NTG and her daughter (MTG) come to Memory & Movement Charlotte to address the children's concerns over their mother's sadness and poor decision-making.

MTG: She has short-term memory deficits and has become reclusive. She has not been the same since Dad died and things are only getting worse. We have begged her to move closer to one of us but she refuses to leave the house she shared with my Dad. It is actually a shrine to him, with everything exactly where it was when he collapsed in the den. She has gained 30 pounds. She claims that it no longer matters. We know she has fallen on several occasions and fear she is drinking too much wine. She has alienated all her friends with the incessant talk of my father and when challenged becomes angry. The house is a mess and her diet consists of chocolate, chips and Chardonnay."

We take a careful history, perform a neuropsychiatric test (perfect score), depression screen and loneliness screen (both positive). Imaging of the brain with an MRI was normal for age.

MTG: Could this be some sort of strange dementia? I have been reading about frontal-temporal dementia where memory is OK but behavior is out of control. She has pushed everyone away, including her children. We are out of bullets. We need your help.

CHE: No, this is not dementia but it is having the same effect. This is a grief reaction that has turned pathological in its intensity and dominance. We are always involved with patients and caregivers dealing with grief reactions. Each is different depending on the underlying relationship and the details of the decline and death.

MTG: We expected trouble early on with my mother. She was devoted to Dad and finally had him solely to herself and then he suddenly was gone. How is this different from a typical response to the death of a spouse?

CHE: I use a metaphor to describe how this works. Your dad now lives in a room in your mother's brain. Since his death, your mom lives in that room. Everything triggers memories of their lives together. In this case, your mother probably went around the house speaking to your dad.

MTG: We thought that was normal at the time.

CHE: It was. Maybe a little odd, but not way out. She felt calm and safe in that room. When distracted or forced out of that room, she became anxious.

MTG: We saw it. She would not leave the house, was tearful and sad all the time. She was up all night sitting in the den where he died. When we encouraged her to get out or see friends, we were confronted with anger, which was out of character for her. She always had a cute personality, never missed the funny part. We never saw that sense of humor again even when a situation would arise that was funny along with sad.

CHE: So in a normal grief reaction, the survivor begins to spend more time out of that room. The demands of life begin to creep in and there is a craving for the attention of family and friends. Slowly the realization forms that there is a life ahead for me. The sense of humor returns. Attention is focused on the future and the adaptation to new realities.

In my counseling sessions following the death of a patient, I stress one crucial point with the surviving caregiver. In this case, it pertains to the room in her brain where her husband resides. I prepare her for the emotions and often anxiety that will come over her every time she enters that room. "You will go in there less and less as life goes on, but every time you go in there, there will be emotion. This is a good thing. It will attach you to him forever, the best memories and the sad ending. You don't have to fear that you will lose him in the coming years, he will always be right there waiting."

The "room in the brain" metaphor serves two purposes:

1. It addresses the pain associated with "moving on" and reassures her that the lost love will in some way always be there.
2. It prepares her for the feelings, good and bad, that will be elicited by those memories. If she knows they are coming, she will be less likely to avoid them and less anxious when they arrive.

MTG: Dr. Edwards, those insights are great for the normal grievers. But we are nowhere close to any normal reaction to anything. Explain what has happened to my mother and is there anything we can do to pull her out of his dive?

CHE: Sorry. But I did want you to get some idea about normal grieving before we get to your mom's situation. I am going to continue with the room metaphor. Even after 7 years, she is still locked in that room. She has canonized your dad and no one, not even her children, can be allowed to share this place. No one has permission to speak about him without making her angry.

MTG: Yes, I have seen that and so have my brothers.

CHE: His death, the suddenness and pain, have resulted in PTSD (post-traumatic stress disorder) coupled with overwhelming anxiety about a future without him.[2] In response to these fears, she has stopped living. Her actions say, "If he is not with me, I don't want to play." Her grief reaction is an obsession with his life and death. The destructive behavior and indifferent response to drinking and the falls is in the "What difference does it make?" column.

MTG: You got it. Now what can we do? She refuses to have any help in the house. No one but she can enter the temple. She will not leave Rock Hill to visit any of us. Do we have any options?

CHE: She is making it tough on you and me. If she will take it, I would start with a medication to help with anxiety and obsessions. If the anxiety and obsession wane, it will help with the anger. I would start low but increase steadily until we get an effect. We need to try again to have help come in to ensure that she is calm, safe and clean. I have to know that she is taking the medicine as prescribed. I will have several counseling sessions with her in the next weeks to address alcohol, driving, medications and social engagement. I would suggest frequent visits from each of the children in the near future.

I wish I could end the profile with an acceptable outcome. But I can't. NTG never allowed us to help her. She continued with the destructive behavior. She broke her hip on one of the falls. Her lack of purpose undermined her rehabilitation. She now lives in assisted living in a retirement center. The obsession with her late husband has never gone away.

Ω

I want to close this discussion with observations on the loss of a loved one. The reason is that if one lives long enough, deep into the *late fragment*, loss of someone dear is almost certain.

I am involved with caregivers after the patient has died. This often involves a short counseling session or phone call to make sure we are on the right track. On occasion, when we are not on the right track, it evolves into more counseling sessions. Those subsequent sessions follow certain patterns that I want to share.

Early after the death of the patient, caregivers struggle with guilt. Strangely, the individuals who have been the most dedicated and provided the highest level of care suffer the most guilt. They are plagued by the times they were impatient or became angry. In this setting, it is imperative that caregivers are reassured that those lapses are universal. This simply indicates that we are all human and, on occasion, will run out of patience and compassion.

The antidote to these feelings of failure is to point out that the patient had a great life with a negative twist at the end. Equal to that is emphasizing the exemplary care the person provided often under trying circumstances. I assure the individual that in time these raw, painful memories will be replaced by ones of better times. I make them tell me a story of a "magic" time in the relationship and encourage them to think of that episode daily.

When this method is not successful, the well-being of the survivor is in jeopardy. The forces that come to bear are formidable and pervasive. They have the capacity and potential to ruin lives. How do we prevent that?

First, let's understand what happens in the brain to allow the abnormal grief reaction to alter a person's enjoyment of life and the connection to others forever. The loss of the loved one is obviously sad and emotionally traumatic to the survivor. Life has irrevocably changed. The future is uncertain. The specter of life without this partner and the certainty (in their mind) of perpetual loneliness results in unbearable anxiety. The human brain will divert this painful uneasiness into an obsession. The real damage occurs with the reaction to the obsession, which is a compulsion. The compulsion becomes evident in excessive time spent with dominant, repetitive thoughts of the lost loved one. When the survivor is living in the shadow of the lost loved ones, they are calm. When they move away from the shadow, they are anxious. They want to be in the shadow forever.

How do we break this cycle of isolation and uneasiness?

There are a myriad of counseling techniques with varied successes. My approach is to try and make the individual aware of the unintended consequences of the obsession with the lost partner. In our experience, abnormal grief reactions overwhelmingly involve the loss of spouses and are more common in women. Difficult situations often involve a setting with no children or in second marriages where the children are not related to the survivor. Loneliness is enhanced in these situations.

The major theme in my counseling sessions is "turn toward the living." The living are usually children but they can be extended family. I make the point that the children have lost a father or mother and are also hurting. Families that share the grief experience recover sooner, and there is less chance of an unhealthy outcome.

A critical element is the children understanding the surviving parent's depth of loss. A normal grief reaction requires time for all involved. But it will be much longer for the surviving spouse. Initially, the survivor spends an inordinate amount of time consumed by the loss. We have already introduced the metaphor, the survivor living in the room in the brain where memories of the lost spouse live. When they are in that room, approaches must be light and respectful. Getting back to normal is the goal. But for the survivor, there is no normal to get back to. That part of their life is gone. Family contact and, when appropriate, family outings are a start to establishing new norms. Once the survivor realizes that love and relevance is assured in this new life, the uneasiness ebbs. Smiles return. We are on the right track.

Abnormal grief reactions are a major landmine in the *late fragment*. They are more common than reported and surprisingly common in caregivers. They are treatable but persistence is the key. Early attempts at connecting with a survivor are often rebuffed. Building a new life alone will be painful. Better to live in that room in my brain with my obsession. Medication can help. But love and understanding work better. Don't give up.

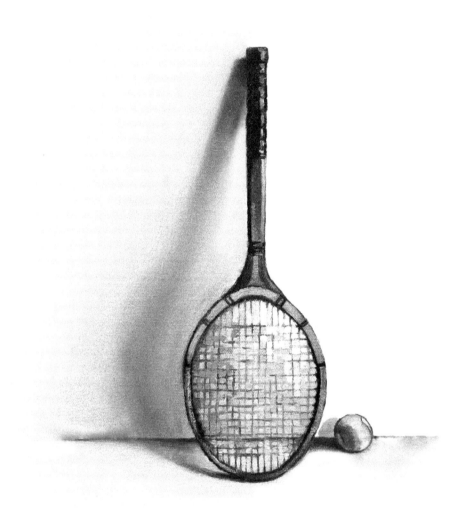

9
Unrealistic Expectations

People can cry much easier than they can change.

James Baldwin

A subtle but crucial theme in this book is how our brain plays tricks on us. These tricks, these illusions, serve a vital purpose in allowing us to function in an uncertain world. Let me show you what I mean.

Example No. 1. If every possible disaster that could befall us is front and center in our thoughts, we would be paralyzed by fear. But the prefrontal cortex, the region that conducts the human brain, allows us to function by altering our perceptions of reality. It suppresses unwelcome outcomes so that we can move through life with a minimum of dread. We want this. We need this.

Example No. 2. The prefrontal cortex works with hope to increase our expectations for the future. We have high hopes, but the actuality never goes that high. When these dashed hopes involve the size of an ice cream cone, the impact is inconsequential. But when it involves the nuts and bolts of life—when it allows one to misread situations that prevents rational responses to important events—harm to all involved can result. The damage can be consequential, even catastrophic.

Ω

Page Mauldin, 82, has been married to her husband Spence for 57 years. They lived in Salisbury, N.C., for their entire marriage. They raised three children there. Spence, 84, was a cardiologist.

Three years ago, they moved to Chapel Hill, N.C., to live in a retirement community. Spence had attended University of North Carolina. They both had the feeling that the timing and choice of the facility was perfect. The children noted that their dad was quieter and mildly forgetful over Christmas and suggested they seek an evaluation at Memory & Movement Charlotte.

They arrive a few minutes late. The patient is dressed in a coat with no tie. He is thin and athletic. He stands when I enter and meets me with a huge smile. We have met before in his role as a cardiologist and mine as a heart surgeon. He recounts the many patients he sent to Charlotte for surgery. He is socially adept and warm. He jokes, "I would rather be in front of you with a heart problem." He then lowers his head and diverts his eyes. "I am here because my wife and children think I am no longer sharp. I hope you can convince me otherwise."

"Spence," I say, "my wife and children think the same about me. I will have your back on this."

His wife appears much younger than her age. Her hair is short and white. Her face is youthful. She is dressed simply. She, too, is socially adept and greets me with a smile.

We initially meet with the couple together but only the patient can speak. We learn that the patient has a history of hypertension and elevated cholesterol. Only recently has the hypertension been treated aggressively. He states that he is aware of memory loss and that he has lost confidence in social situations. I ask the question: "On any given morning, you wake up and say 'This is going to be a great day because I get to do this,' what is *this?*"

Spence: I'm not sure now. I look forward to seeing family and the grandchildren but things have changed. When we first moved, I looked forward to being with my old Carolina mates, playing golf, gin rummy and spending time together. I am not doing this as much now. I'm not sure why.

CHE: Are you happy in Chapel Hill?

Spence: I was at first. I'm not sure now. I think Page thinks we made a bad decision to come here.

Spence has been tested. I have reviewed his brain imaging. He has MCI (mild cognitive impairment) that has affected his short-term memory. The MRI shows "white matter changes" slightly more advanced than would be predicted from age alone. This is the result of the vascular disease from inadequately treated hypertension. At this point, this is not dementia. The downside is that 70% of patients with MCI go on to develop dementia. The depression screen was surprisingly positive.

We separate patient from spouse and I spend 20 to 30 minutes with the wife. I explain that his memory issues are the result of hypertension and how important it is that he takes the two blood pressure meds as prescribed.

CHE: Spence mentioned that you think you may have made a bad decision moving to Chapel Hill. Are you not happy in your present situation?

Page: I don't want to say I am unhappy, but I can't make the jump to happy, if that makes any sense.

CHE: Expand on that. Is Spence right when he says you regret the decision to move to Chapel Hill?

Page: Let me start by describing what we left. We lived in Salisbury for more than 50 years. We raised our children there, grew old with our friends. It is not unusual that I would miss it.

CHE: What are the things you miss the most?

Page: I miss my church friends, my garden club friends, my tennis buddies and I miss playing tennis. I miss our couple friends and all the stuff we used to do. We had a great life that I cherished. I left all that behind. It's not that people have not been nice. We have made friends and do things. It's just different.

CHE: Tell me about your friends back in Salisbury. Has time stood still there and all those activities are still going on without you?

Page: I can't say that. Our two closest couple friends have also left for retirement communities, one in Pinehurst and the other in Richmond, Va. The garden club has folded. It is all so sad.

CHE: Page, if you returned to live in Salisbury tomorrow, would any of your old life still be intact?

Page: No, I suppose not.

CHE: What about the tennis? The facility in Chapel Hill has tennis courts. Why aren't you playing with new friends there?

Page: I can't play tennis anymore. I have a bad hip and fell trying to play. I can't even play pickleball. Every time I see other residents playing tennis, I feel sad, often teary.

CHE: What I am hearing from you is that the move is responsible for the loss of many of the pleasurable aspects of your life. You have not been able to duplicate the idyllic situation that you had for five decades. The loss of all that has resulted in a sadness with life in general.

Page: I am not an unhappy person. I am just saying this was not what I expected when we moved. It is different and I have not been able to accept it.

CHE: I know you are aware that the life you had before the move is gone. You did not move away from an ideal situation. The ideal situation moved away from you.

Page: I just can't seem to get past it. Now Spence is beginning to have some memory issues and the whole thing is falling apart. We never quarreled in our marriage, but recently we are both irritable. I have been impatient with him. He seems to be sensitive to any comment I make. He has never been a dependent person, actually the opposite. He now seems to be tethered to me. He has lost interest in golf and going with his friends. We are in trouble. I hope you can help us.

CHE: I am going to speak with Spence. After I do that, we will get back together.

I walk next door and examine Spence. The blood pressure is too high, 155/90. We will communicate with his primary care doctor to address it. Otherwise, the exam is negative. The MOCA score (neuropsychiatric test) is 27/30. The deficits were down 2 out of 5 on short-term memory and 1 down on math. For his age, this is a good score.

CHE: Spence, do you think you made a mistake moving to Chapel Hill? It seems that life was changing in Salisbury long before you left.

Spence: One of the reasons we considered leaving was the fact that our two closest couple friends had moved to retirement communities far from Salisbury. She cannot play tennis anymore and this has increased her dissatisfaction with the status quo. She seems to dismiss all this.

CHE: Are you aware when your memory lets you down, when you are no longer on your A game?

Spence: Names give me trouble, especially in the dining room. I am not as good on the computer and I write everything down. But overall I think I'm doing OK. What I'm not doing OK with is Page. She has the obsession that the move ruined her life. I don't know what she expected, but for her it is far from the reality. I think perhaps she is disappointed in me. I don't look forward to getting up in the morning. It is just another day trying to reason with her about something she is unreasonable about.

We come back together.

CHE: First, I am glad you have come and we have reconnected. We have some work to do before we get back the life that preceded the move. I am going to start with a sentence that comes from my first book, *Much Abides*. It says, "Mourning the loss of what you had is too easy and it prevents us from the hard work of making a life out of what is left."

Spence, you don't have Alzheimer's disease or any type of dementia. We do have mild memory loss but it doesn't seem to affect your everyday life. This is called Mild Cognitive Impairment. The move, the mild memory loss, and your perception that Page is unhappy has resulted in situational depression. It will require treatment. It will take a while, but we can make this better.

Page: Wait. It is unfair to pin all this on me. We both have struggled with adapting to this new life. Every day I am reminded of what we left behind. It seems out of proportion to what others in Chapel Hill deal with. I came here with high hopes that we could duplicate the happiness we shared in Salisbury. It is unrealistic to assume I would not be bitterly disappointed. Yes, I admit it. I am angry. I feel that if I am not mad, I will have given up. I mean, given up on being happy.

We separate again and I am alone with Page.

CHE: Page, no one is "pinning" this on you. I would like to share my early observations here and offer a few suggestions that might get us pointed in the right direction. Are you up for this?

Page: We came for help. Yes.

CHE: You are working under two illusions that have deceived you and thrown you off your game. One is rather easy to overcome. The second is a universal struggle. In this situation, the two are connected at the source. Navigating this impasse will require desire, wisdom and fortitude. You have the potential to navigate all three.

    An illusion is something that deceives us by producing a false impression, a deceit. The first illusion that we need to face is the impact of the move. It goes something like this. "For whatever reason, Spence and I thought it time to drastically change our lives by moving into a retirement center. We impulsively left almost a perfect life—friends, church, activities and tennis. We had the unreal expectation that we could recreate our former life in this new setting."

The first part of the illusion is that you can return to Salisbury and resume that idyllic life. The second part of the illusion is that your new setting lacks the potential to provide happiness and the connectivity you previously enjoyed. The move is now an obsession that dominates your thoughts and moods every day. A third and major part of the illusion is thinking that your unhappiness and obsession only affects you and has no impact on those who love and depend on you.

You are a smart lady. I know on some level that you know the life in Salisbury is gone forever. The people and feelings of connectedness are no longer in place. You would be returning to a home that is no longer your home. You know that.

Page: If this is so obvious to you, why is it not obvious to me? Why is it always front and center in my brain?

CHE: Now we are getting to it. The answer is that the first illusion allows you to avoid coming face to face with the second illusion. The second illusion is that your life will go on unimpeded. Aging will not be a factor and you won't have to contend with your inability to play tennis, your husband's fragile memory and being forced out of your comfort zone by time and physical decline. By focusing on the move, you avoided the pain that comes with confronting the irrevocable and certain consequences of aging lives. It was easier to be angry at the move than despondent and anguished over the real forces affecting you.

Page: Is it really that helpless?

CHE: No. But it can't be solved until we face it.

Page: How do I do that?

CHE: You've already started when you said, "I am not giving up." That defiance is the crucial element we need to make this work.

Page: Explain that to me.

CHE: You've already drawn lines you refuse to cross, certain declines you refuse to surrender to. You have just drawn them in the wrong place. We want the defiance. But we want it placed where it can dissolve this anger and isolation.

Page: I am angry and I feel alone. But I'm not sure I follow what you are getting at.

CHE: Now that we have established the real enemy—not the move but the attacks on us from the passage of time—we can use the weapons we possess more strategically. You have drawn the lines of defense too close to you. You have not included your husband, and he is suffering from the isolation and anger. I want the defiance to say, "I am going to protect this marvelous man and the two of us will be a formidable team to fight this potential for despair." I want the defiance to say, "My attitude, my perspective can make any situation better and I refuse to let selfish, negative thoughts undermine our struggle." I want the defiance to say, "I have room for new friends that I can connect with to give and receive help when needed." I want the defiance to say, "I realize now that I have to connect with others through our shared vulnerabilities, not with the remorse of things I have lost."

Page: Wow. You are setting some high bars for me.

CHE: We will get there with small, certain steps. Let's start by being positive and sharing that positivity with your husband. I think you may be shocked at how quickly the anger and irritability respond.

Page: I get it. Whether I can do it is a different question.

CHE: Just start by controlling the spin when you talk to yourself. No negative, only positive.

One month later:

Page: I should be furious at you. You called me selfish, angry, delusional and implied even more sinister attributes. I had always considered myself a good person.

CHE: Our brains don't like to confront pain.

Page: It was painful. I had gotten into a trap and I could see no way out. It wasn't until I realized that my anger was hurting those around me and, more than anything, was hurting *me* that I started back. I'm not completely there but I am more positive. The daily spats are gone. We are both thinking ahead and trying to connect with the life here in Chapel Hill.

CHE: I am proud of you, especially for not firing me.

Page: Don't think you are out of the woods yet!!

Unrealistic expectations and their unreliable partners, high hopes, are especially destructive in the later stages of life. The fact that we are always in the neighborhood of loss and decline makes the consequences of losing hope more significant. Understanding how and why our brains foster the creation of illusions and the sinister impact they have on our well-being, will keep us on guard.

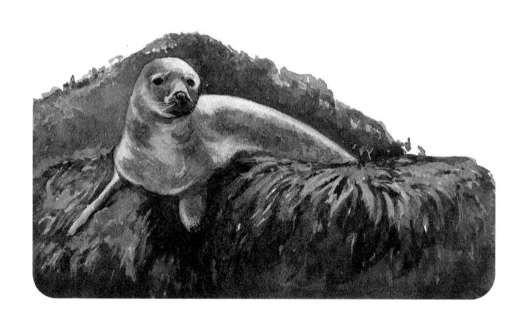

10
Illusions:
Some We Need, Some We Don't

EARL

In Sitka, because they are fond of them
People have named the seals. Every seal
is named Earl because they are killed one
after another by the orca, the killer
whale: seal bodies tossed left and right
into the air. "At least he didn't get
Earl," someone says. And sure enough
after a time, that same friendly,
bewhiskered face bobs to the surface.
It's Earl again. Well, how else are you
to live except by denial, by some
palatable fiction, some little song to
sing while the inevitable, the black and
white blindsiding fact, comes hurtling
toward you out of the deep?

Louis Jenkins

In my practice caring for people with dementia, I deal with delusions and hallucinations every day. Alzheimer's disease, vascular dementia, Parkinson's disease and all the spinoffs attack the perceptions of reality in the brain. A question we ask our families on every visit is, "Have you seen any breaks with reality?" They are that common.

Memory lapses become easy for families and caregivers to manage. You supply the answer to the repetitive question and move on. Breaks with reality are more distressing. They don't border on crazy—they *are* crazy. The delusions run the gamut of concern. "Someone has taken my stuff" is not as serious as a patient thinking, "My spouse is having an affair," or misthinking—"I don't live here. I live in a place exactly like this but not here." That last one triggers wandering. These are catastrophic, pathological upheavals in the minds of patients whose lives have been taken over by a disease.

This stuff can't apply to our lives, right? We are sane, sound, no tricks of the mind here.

Hold on. Let's go deeper.

Insights and valuable lessons—information we need to understand our own realities—come from the edges of this human drama. When I treated individuals with dementia by day and wrote about the demands of those living long lives at night, I saw an interplay. A sliver of common ground. Questions arose. Do the illusions of dementia, that craziness, have anything to teach those who consider themselves sane and whole? Would knowing how this cerebral deception works help me understand the confusion and weariness I feel at times?

The answer is a resounding YES. The more I thought about the fragile reality of those living on the edge, the more I became aware of how fragile our realities are, especially in the *late fragment*, and why.

First, let's define illusions and delusions and why it is important to understand their impact.

- **Illusion.** The condition of being deceived by erroneous perceptions or beliefs.
- **Delusion.** A false fixed belief.

An *illusion*, the denial of reality, requires our brains to play tricks on us. We are beguiled into believing what is real is not and allowing false perceptions to explain the reality. Before we get into how the brain does this, we need to explain why it happens. This is where the tricks start, with our brains and anxiety.

Anxiety is defined as painful uneasiness. Humans from birth are hopelessly enmeshed with this uneasiness. They are acutely aware of its presence and will go to great lengths to make it stop. The brains of anxious humans have become adept over millions of years in dealing with these unnerving sensations by ignoring them. We delude ourselves into thinking that there is no need to be nervous. There is no danger when rationally we know there is great danger. This is the illusion we need.

Louis Jenkins in the poem "Earl" that I shared at the start of this chapter describes it perfectly. "How else are we to live except by denial, by some palatable fiction, some little song to sing while the inevitable, the black and white blindsiding fact, comes hurtling toward us..." The image of the orca blindsiding us is too graphic, the carnage too violent, to imagine. That's where the "little song" comes in to distract us. Obviously being attacked by a killer whale is an exaggeration (except for Earl). But it *does* demonstrate the need for the illusion.

The deception occurs in the frontal lobe of our brains in the vicinity of the anxiety that demands the illusion.[1] Without the ability to tamp down fears and forebodings, the majority of us would be paralyzed in the face of life's everyday dangers. A more modern, reasonable example of this process would be driving at high speed down a two-lane highway in heavy traffic. One has to sing a "little song" that says everyone driving toward me is a safe and cautious person with excellent eyesight and reactions. I am comfortable with them being a few feet to the side of me, coming at high speed. None of these fellow travelers would ever drink alcohol, use drugs or drive impaired.

We know this assessment to be false. But by deceiving ourselves, danger is dimmed and feelings of safety are summoned. The illusion that I will be fine allows us to function surrounded by sinister threats. Without this process in the frontal lobe, we would all still be huddled in a prehistoric cave too frightened to venture out. This illusion, the ability to ignore elements of reality that cause anxiety and fear, has been basic to survival and progress since humans first evolved. We need this illusion. It has served us well.

But there is a hitch. A patient of mine, Gretchen Ames, is a perfect illustration of how the hitch works. Gretchen, 76, has struggled with anxiety her entire life. "I was born with it," she says. Her first marriage was marked by abuse, both verbal and, on one occasion, physical. Anxiety was accelerated beyond tolerance. She broke from it and eventually remarried a kind, gentle man who "made me forget the past and the trauma buried there. We have been together for thirty-six years."

During a recent visit she shared, "Memories of my first marriage have come back with vengeance. Nothing in my life has changed, Why now? Is there an explanation?"

She is dealing with the hitch. The frontal lobe is the conductor of the entire brain. It is where we are civilized, set social boundaries, and solve simple problems. It is not fully developed in humans until the mid-20s, which explains the relative absence of judgment in teenagers and young adults. Despite being the dominant domain in the human brain, it is the site of the most aggressive effects of aging. Atrophy (shrinkage) of the frontal lobe approaches 0.25% to 0.5% per year after a person reaches the late 20s, far surpassing the effect of age on other domains. The math is simple. Twenty-eight-year-olds today who retire at 65 will have lost 10 to 20% of the size of their frontal lobes. The exact effect of this atrophy on brain function is not predictable. But it is significant. [2]

What is also predictable is the decline in the ability of the frontal lobe to control anxiety and divert us from the surrounding dangers. It follows that aging adults are more anxious in the face of travails then when they were younger and confronting the same circumstances. Older individuals are more susceptible to triggers that reignite painful memories thought to be forgotten. The necessary illusion that we are safe in this ominous world lets us down and leaves us nervous.

The aging Gretchen Ames is struggling with all of this. The fact that she has harbored high levels of anxiety throughout her life has provided a perfect culture for her frontal lobe curbs to be overwhelmed. She again is being marred by these crippling memories. This is more evidence of the effectiveness of the illusion and the destructive forces that arise in its absence.

The second trick I want to uncover is the relationship of the human brain to time. The fact that our brains often do not effectively sense the passage of time causes countless misconceptions over a lifetime. The consequences of these misconceptions are magnified in the *late fragment*.

In shorter intervals we need the sun or a device to measure time. In longer intervals our eyes see its effect when looking at others or examining our image in the mirror. The ears hear it when we note the changes in timbre in the voice of aging individuals. We feel it in our joints which become stiffer and crankier with the physical demands of age. Strangely, the brain records only the present moment. It can remember the past and anticipate the future, but the sensation, the awareness that time is passing is indifferent.

When we are aware of time, it is not pleasant. We become aware of time when there is a deadline, a timed task or we are late. In every instance that the brain is aware of the elapsing of time, there is tension. The closer we are to running out of time, the stakes rise. Anxiety elevates into agitation. Agitation crashes into panic. All of it is unpleasant, unwanted.

Understanding how our brains process time is critical to assigning value to intervals in our lives. Grades in school, time spent in college, sports careers and actual careers are predictable phases of life. Each of these critical intervals has a ceremony, a ritual to mark the end of this time. Graduations, final games and retirement parties are signs that life has moved on. These rituals also serve to refocus us on the next interval, a new phase, the future.

The problem arises in the other spans of time when no limits are in place. Without the limits, without artificial structures within a span of time, there is no urgency. There is no signal to warn us that "this is over." The value of the time and our effectiveness in that frame drops precipitously.

This is especially true for individuals in the late stages of life. The presence of the fatigue of age and the absence of palpable goals and loss of will to attain those goals combine to discount the value of time. After retirement, there are no ceremonies to mark an achievement, no rituals to refocus us on the future.

Oh, wait. There *is* one ceremony that awaits us all. But unlike previous celebrations, the enthusiasm for this appointment is muted. Our brains have prevented us from thinking about this drab day. When an inkling of this certainty enters our awareness, anxiety rushes in to divert our thoughts and trick us into thinking that, in this one case, I just might beat the odds.

All this preamble leads to The Grand Delusion. I AM GOING TO LIVE FOREVER. *This* illusion we don't need.

Once again, anxiety works against us, this time for keeps. If I will always be here, there is no need to account for anything. There will always be time to make amends, to set the record straight. No words are needed to support the idiocy of this strategy.

The way a crow
Shook down on me
The dust of snow
From a hemlock tree

Has given my heart
A change of mood
And saved some part
Of a day I rued.
— Robert Frost —

When Frost wrote this poem, he was at the same point we are now, trying to preserve the value of each segment of our lives. The "dust of snow from a hemlock tree" is a premonition of his death. It is a day he rued. The change of mood has the possibility to make him aware of the limits of his time on earth. This awareness could be the beginning of changing perspectives that make this last phase of life, something he feared, come alive.

It seems an inadequate metaphor. But the contemplation of one's death, the buzzer at the end, could bring the time preceding it into focus. This focus could be the trigger to allow everything of value to crystallize, to take on urgency. If the goal is to be relevant and involved, it has to include this step.

Why would anyone resist this process? It seems natural that all of us would want to do some soul-searching toward the end. Again, asking the right questions and demanding answers leads us in the right direction. Am I on the right track? Do the people I love know I love them? Do I have issues to resolve before I go? Do I have a legacy? If so, what is it? It seems simple. Certainly everyone would want to think about these things.

Anxiety keeps raising its sinister head, even late. When we must answer for actions, outcomes, shortcomings and failures from a lifetime, the accounting is painful but necessary. It is also liberating. Once we bring these regrets into focus and relive the experience with the goal of forgiving others and ourselves, the anxiety tied to the memories disappears.

So what's the trick and why does our brain do it? The human brain is magnificent at avoiding pain and uneasiness linked to the past. Memories that are stored with emotion are cordoned off by a wall of painful uneasiness. When we go near them, think about them, and try to relive them, we are stopped. The brain says, "Do you really want to experience this again? It is going to hurt. Let's do this another time."

This forces us to carry around the anxiety from a lifetime of the things that didn't work out, that hurt. We are aware of the temporary calm that results from avoiding these painful places. But we are prevented from resolving the internal conflicts that arise from them. This trick, this avoidance, relegates us to perpetual anxiety which undermines the calm we crave late in life. When time begins to run out and regrets mount, the ability to resolve those regrets becomes an essential element to happiness itself.

Every life has some regrets, some small, some huge. Forgiveness—forgiving others and especially forgiving ourselves—is a crucial step that results in our finally securing a release from painful memories.

The number of tricks our brains are capable of playing on us are legion. Some are inconsequential. Others, like the two I have covered, can change lives. The first step is to acknowledge that you are anxious.

A question follows. "What am I anxious about?" The *late fragment* can provide answers that have evaded us and every wise man who ever lived.

Take heart. There is peace hidden behind anxiety. A place of calm lies just beyond the horizon. To reach it requires facing off against feelings of insecurity and uneasiness. Reliving difficult moments. Mustering the courage to ask the question and then answering it for yourself.

We all deserve one of those "Lifetime Achievement Awards" that are given to celebrities in the motion picture business. Not every movie they made or role they played was award-winning but, overall, it was pretty good. Envision yourself walking off the stage with the award given to you by your peers and thinking that you are being rewarded for your role in real life, not the movies. You were not perfect, but you accomplished some marvelous feats.

It is time we turned the tables and played a few tricks back on our brains using the newfound confidence that was always there.

Part III
Directive

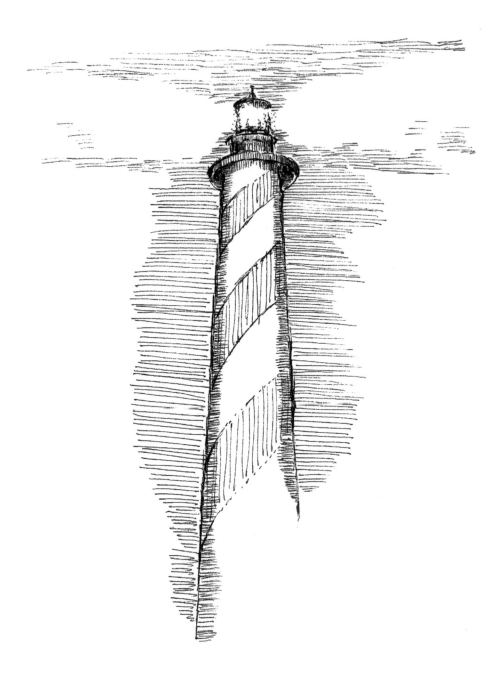

11
Resilience

Your mind will give to you exactly what you put in it.

James Joyce

In the introduction, I stated that I would never have started this book if I hadn't thought I could deliver on the promise of making this *late fragment* not only tolerable but worthy of the life that preceded it. We have arrived at Part 3, the final section. It's time to deliver on that promise.

Everything written so far has been to set up these final chapters. I have shared why I chose to write this book and the struggles that complicated that intent. I've acknowledged the bond with my aging colleagues that was born out of those struggles.

I have covered the ultimate goal, which is to understand the unique demands of long lives and to outwit the factors that threaten the potential of this precious interval. I've told you why this time tacked on to the end is decisive in ensuring the significance of the whole. The reasons why this is hard have been catalogued and the landmines identified. We now know who is in the *late fragment* and why.

Tennyson preceded us here. He warned us that time and fate had weakened us. He reminded us of our heroic hearts and strong wills which once moved heaven and earth. My role is to connect those heroic hearts and strong wills to the challenges that late life presents and, once again, turn them loose.

What strengths are left and what is the source of that strength? Individual character is the basic element we carry through life. Good or bad, we have done "stuff" and our personal stories are the source of strength in this late phase. We've had successes, the result of dedication, skill and hard work. Equally important are the survival instincts, the fortitude and grit we drew strength from when we encountered hard times or gut-wrenching setbacks.

These truths are eternal. But the character traits that are in play are different at different times in our lives. Courage is always needed, but it takes on a different look in the *late fragment*. Let's take a look at what courage looks like in an 89-year-old retired high school English teacher.

Ω

Meet Evelyn Brooks. She never married. Her life was her students. She was 25 when she began teaching English at a Charlotte, N.C. high school. Forty years later, she walked out of that same school knowing she had changed the lives of thousands of her students. Revered is the operative word. She was hard but often remarked that demanding a great deal from students resulted in their realizing they were capable of achieving a great deal.

She lived next door to her sister, a high school history teacher, in a small house one block from the school.

Four years ago, she lost her sister to heart disease.

"You must understand how close we were," she says. "She was a vital part of every day of my life. We were both too strong-willed to live together but we were oddly inseparable. We shared every activity, almost every thought. I had never been away from her. The pain was too much. I thought I would die.

"But I didn't. It took time, but I slowly made it back. One poem that I taught every year kept repeating itself to me. The more despair I felt, the more it was there. It was John Milton's 'On Blindness.' The opening lines…

> When I consider how my light is spent,
> ere half my days in this dark world and wide,
> And that one Talent which is death to hide
> Lodged with me useless…[1]

"I would remind my students that Milton wrote *Paradise Lost* after losing his sight. I would describe him dictating the lines to his daughter. After losing his sight, he thought that one talent—his poetic genius—was lodged within him, useless. I would explain that God demands we use our talents. I wanted them to see that great things may be done in one's life even in the face of crippling adversity.

"I finally made the connection. Milton was talking directly to me. I made it back, slowly at first, but I heard his voice every day and finally, I recovered."

Evelyn created a new life out of nieces, nephews, former students, fellow teachers. Daily deep dives into her readings sustained her.

I use her story to make a point about the changing face of character traits with aging. We miscalculate when we think of courage, bravery and survival in terms of battlefields and warriors. I maintain that Miss Brooks showed unrivaled courage and tenacity when she escaped from the despair of losing the most important person in her life. Age will test us all. The role of "warrior" seems to fit this 84-year-old retired English teacher.

Miss Brooks had a distinctive teaching style. Every class started with quotes from literature. She would stand in front of the class and begin to recite the passage and the class would immediately pick up the cadence. The quotes came from Coleridge, Frost, Milton, Shakespeare, A.E. Houseman, Pope, Thomas Grey, and others.

The purpose of this ritual was to etch these famous sayings into the brains of her students forever. She taught her students to love the literature—the poems, plays and novels. She wanted them to know the characters, their stories, and the universal truths revealed in them. Miss Brooks's intent was to provide a richness to the fabric of her students' lives and, if needed, to serve as source of light if lives darkened.

The strengths that she used to achieve this effect were dedication, preparation, concern for each student, and a compelling individualism that made it all work. In her current situation, except for the individualism, the very attributes that were critical to making Miss Brooks an outstanding teacher are no longer needed. Sadly, now there is no one to be dedicated to, no one to prepare lessons for, no one to inspire with literature that will enrich their lives. Surely this amazing woman with such a strong sense of herself and a track record of survival can tap into deeper traits that can sustain her through to the end.

The rituals, techniques, and dedication she displayed for her students were deep traits. But they were not the core constituents of her character. They were strategies for the role she chose to play, that of a teacher.

If Evelyn Brooks had chosen another career, one can imagine a different set of strategies would have been held just as dear. Some might describe them as necessary attributes grafted on to core values of character. But those strategies, those attributes, cannot sustain us. Having been a successful banker, lawyer or teacher cannot sustain us in the *late fragment*. That success is in the past. Gone. It is a beguiling illusion to think that what happened once upon a time has the power to match the ravages of time.

Two eternal elements are crucial to staying relevant late in life. The first is **resilience**. The dictionary defines resilience as being resourceful or flexible in changing circumstances. But I've come to realize that resilience in the *late fragment* is better understood as resistance bordering on defiance. Resilience to me, especially late resilience, is a struggle to preserve my dignity and my intellectual independence, and not to surrender to loss or victimhood. We need to be flexible in accepting the realities of long lives. But underlying that must be a resolve, a resistance, a defiance to losing our souls in this time of decline. We do not lose our places in this world because we are old.

The second eternal element is **authenticity**. I define it as the avenue to my true self. It is saying, "Before I go, I want everyone to know who I am, what I think, and especially why I think my life has been worthwhile. Remember this when I am gone."

My reason for including authenticity is to stress the fact that no one who has ever lived has your DNA and life experiences. You are unique. You are the author of a story that is going to be told one time. Just because it is late in the story does not mean that you are done. By coming at it from this angle, I hope to recharge some batteries or rekindle some fading embers. We may have some potential impact, some tread left on our tires.

Back to Miss Brooks. She prevailed (she would love this word) until a fall forced her into assisted living at a retirement center. Ironically, like her muse Milton, her eyesight diminished to the point she could no longer read. The fractured hip limited her mobility and required a walker. The light was fading. What was left?

Dylan Thomas told Evelyn to "rage against the dying of the light" and she did.[2] She kept a rigid schedule and forced herself to walk outside with her walker even in sketchy weather. She listened to books on tape every day. Her joy came from the association with a group of retired teachers who listen to the classics on tape several afternoons a week. She lived long enough that some of her students were in the same facility. They often visited her. She raged until the end.

She was sustained by knowing her legacy—great stories, poems and plays are a gift to us. They can also provide guidance and even structure to hold on to when we get confused or decline. She can attest to that. She also knew that she would live forever in the lives of her students who will teach their children and grandchildren about the value of literature.

Just as each of us is telling a story, a story that will be told only once, each of us has a legacy to those left behind. It, too, is singular, and emanates from each of our interactions with other humans over a lifetime. The *late fragment* is the perfect setting to examine the legacy being left and to adjust it if need be.

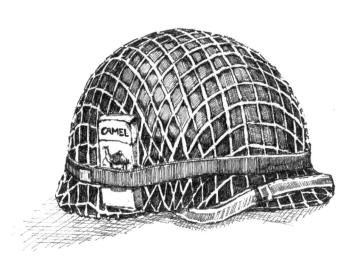

12

Vital Links

At times our own light goes out and is rekindled
by a spark from another person. Each of us
has cause to think with deep gratitude of those
that have lighted the flame within us.

Albert Schweitzer

Allof us are searching for elements to help sustain us later in life. Some are hardware—railings, grab bars, canes, and walkers. They steady us when we stumble or help us up when we fall. But other aids are the ultimate "software"—humans who can understand, listen and guide.

We have just looked at the vital role our own history can play. This is when we rely on ourselves, our personal resilience and core strengths, to push on. But there will be times when the demands and strain are too much and we will need a hand from other humans who know us and care about us. To perceive this need as weakness is insanity. To navigate an entire life, all the curves and cliffs, requires our finding strength and wisdom from anywhere and anyone who has the potential to help. These vital links are mentors. Some are heroes.

A mentor is "one who advises" or "someone who shows the way." One colossal misconception about aging is that wisdom naturally accompanies that aging. In truth, those who have navigated long lives and come away with valuable insight and acumen are rare. If genuine wisdom was as prevalent as many believe, our tendency to go off course or get turned around in our lives would be uncommon. We know that to be untrue.

This simple reality puts those individuals who can guide us and are willing to do so in a sacred place in our lives. Sadly, the longer we live, the number of individuals who can play those roles decline. A majority of them are gone.

This leaves us two options. The first is to search for new influences, new guides. Your most effective mentor, even hero, may be a close friend or right in front of you in a son or daughter. The second option is to reconnect with those who have left this world physically but their influence and advice is still available in the form of memories.

An enjoyable part of my work week is my Wednesday clinic at a retirement center here in Charlotte. My nurse, Shelly, and I see patients and families that mostly are in the *late fragment*. We love our time there. The bonds that have been forged with these individuals are irreplaceable in our lives. We are part of stories moving toward the end and have been allowed to tag along and share this matchless time with them. We are attending a course in human drama that enriches our present lives and prepares us for our time in the same circumstance.

A month ago, a casual interface with a 94-year-old man gave evidence to how this all plays out.

I take a short break around 10 a.m. and go into a library where there is coffee. I usually sit alone for 15 to 20 minutes. On one of these mornings, I see one of my patients sitting at a table.

CHE: Ivan, how are you this morning? You are usually gone by this hour.

Ivan: Hi, Doc. You have caught me at a bad time. I am having a mini pity party this morning. I am off my game.

CHE: Tell me what's going on. Why are you down?

Ivan: As you know, I have coffee with Julie Cook here in the library every morning. We have been friends since boyhood. We are the same age. I start every day with him and have ever since we both arrived here nearly ten years ago. Our wives are gone now. My friendship with Julie was one of the only things that has survived from my previous life. One week ago, he went to the ER with pain in his back and he never came back. It came out of nowhere. This is my first day back at this table where we met every day. (He shakes his head.). I'm just off, that's all.

CHE: I'm sorry about Julie. What a good guy. Everyone is going to miss him.

Ivan: I know. I was just thinking how arbitrary all this is. Here we are the same age. Neither one of us had any major medical issues. Then BOOM! Why not me?

CHE: Can't help you there. The answer to that question is way above my pay grade. I just hate to see you hurting like this.

Ivan: When I see you in the clinic, you always ask me, "What keeps you going? What do you look forward to?" That question is getting harder to answer with each passing day. Not year, but day.

I'm sorry to bore you with all this. I guess I am having trouble even thinking about what life is going to be without my buddy, Julie. He and I were the lone rangers. Everyone else is gone.

CHE: Believe me when I say that you are not boring me. I am impressed that you are up and strong enough to share all this. I know it's hard to even find the words to describe how you feel.

Ivan: I am the end of the line in my family. Anne Marie and I were unable to have children. My sister and my brothers had no children. I guess if I had grandchildren or, now, great-grandchildren that things would be different. I could look at the future with a different spin. For me, there is no future except for what happened to Julie this week.

CHE: Give it time. You may live longer than you think. Life may have a few surprises left.

Ivan: I don't want you to think that I am not grateful for my life. All said and done, I have had a great life. You know what's strange? Now my mind and the memories in it go backward. I spend more time in the past. I see it so clearly. Two people in my life keep coming back, vividly and often. Strangely, the two men, who now are a great source of solace to me in my 90s, both died young.

One is my older brother, Seth. I was three years younger. He was my hero from my first memories. He was a great athlete in every sport and really smart. But that is not what I remember. He was gentle and kind, especially to me. He was never afraid. Knowing what to do and how to do it was instinctive for him. In contrast, I was always afraid.

My father had a stock phrase when describing individuals. They either matched up or they didn't. Seth always matched up. I was never sure I could. Even as a young boy, I would ask "What would Seth do?" It gave me courage to stay strong.

Seth was killed in World War II in the South Pacific during the battle of Peleliu. My family never recovered. A later description of the battle includes a paragraph of his final moments fighting off several Japanese soldiers with his hands. It's only recently that memories of him have been allowed to come back. I suppressed them for many years. They were too painful. For some reason, every detail of him has rushed back and is with me every day.

The second person who has come back to me is my first partner in business, Duncan McDonald. We were best friends, went to college together and early on dreamed of starting a business together. We got off to a great start. The future looked bright.

One day he finished shaving, looked in the mirror and his entire face was a bruise—dark, almost black discoloration. Acute leukemia. He lived three weeks. I spent those three weeks with him. What I remember early was a daily greeting by the bruised face that had become a fuzzy background to a huge smile. The smile never faded. In the first week of his survival, I thought, "Doesn't he understand where this is going?" Surely he can't be this strong, to know and to keep his spirits so high. He would talk about a future he was not part of and warn me about stuff. Well, he *was* that strong. The smile never faded. I can still see it clearly.

Doc, I spend a lot of time with Seth and Duncan these days. They matched up in their test and I am going to match up in mine. I've talked enough. Thanks for your time and ear.

He rose from his seat, stood up tall and resolute. He nodded his head gently toward me, smiled and walked off.

Ω

The process of finding these mentors, these heroes, is not passive. They do not return and sustain us without a sincere, active search. These influences, these sustaining memories, are hidden in remote recesses in our brains. Time and the tumult of lives have obscured the paths to this strength and wisdom. Finding the map to these treasures requires that we realize we need these individuals in our lives again.

In the *late fragment*, the glow from achievement and money is long gone. We are left with the bare bones of life. Lying among these remains are the memories of heroes who at one time got some of all this right. There is warmth and mettle in these vital links, enough to carry us to the end.

13

Accepting New Roles

Relic: *Something that has survived the passage of
time. An object or custom whose original purpose
has disappeared. Anything left over. Remnant.*

It is Thanksgiving, a major gathering for our clan. I am part of a
throng of 20 crammed into one room. This is my family—my
wife, children, grandchildren, nieces, nephews, in-laws and out-
laws. A central conversation is raging that has ignited partisan and
intense responses from every corner of the room. The exact topic
has been lost to me, but it centers on some fad in pop culture and
the predictable reaction from the generations present. Boomers are
appalled, millennials defensive, and Gens X, Y, and Z all over the
place. Shouting, laughter and incredulity break out. The floor is hard
to get, impossible to hold.

I have a point I want to make. I am willing to wait my turn. But
even with raising my voice, my time never comes. The frustration
forces me back to a time when my voice would have had precedent.
It might have been out of respect but this group would have wanted
to hear what I had to say. Though it might have required a significant
level of boldness or even rudeness to be heard, I'd have had my say.

Not today.

Miraculously, my wife, Mary, managed to get everyone's attention (with a soft voice) and began to speak. Leaping into the fray, I interrupted her, and began to speak. She turned to me with mild venom and said (sarcastically), "Oh, pardon me, did the middle of my sentence interrupt the beginning of yours?" (She stole the line from a movie she saw earlier that week.)

This literally brought the house down. The glee was somewhat out of proportion and caused me embarrassment and shame. It prompted a mini-pout. "I'll just keep this point to myself," I thought, pitifully. "They will regret leaving this discussion without my insight."

What it really prompted was a painful replaying of the incident and, in my mind, the asking of several questions. Why did Mary's voice garner the attention that I wanted when my voice was louder and definitely more urgent? Could it be that they were not interested in what my opinion was on this particular subject? Or worse, did they already know what I was going to say?

The answers to these questions weren't coming. I just know it hurt. I was struggling with a minor rejection. "Come on. Shrug it off. Grow up," I said to myself. Then I realized that what I was really fighting off was a premonition of irrelevance. If I can't use my voice to teach, persuade, impress, then I have become inert, incapable of being taken seriously on any subject.

Surely these young people get me. They know I love them and care what they think. I lecture because I know things they are going to need to know. In my life, I have made mistakes, gotten things wrong. I want to prevent them from making the mistakes. I also strongly believe there are universal truths and values that must be transferred to future generations. I can't sit quietly when there is an opportunity to make a vital point.

Why was Mary able to get everyone's attention? I can see that she never lectures or demands the floor. She is curious about all their lives and what is going on in them. The questions she asks and the way she asks them establish trust. They encourage questions to be asked back. The values and opinions are passed seamlessly and effectively—no pomp, no circumstance, no lecture.

As you can see, I had to endure a painful episode to gain a valuable insight. The passage of character traits from generation to generation is best done with a feather rather than a sledgehammer.

I thought I had been humbled enough for one holiday. But a double whammy was in my immediate future.

Be curious, not judgmental.[1]

Ted Lasso

About an hour after the above fiasco, I was sitting alone with Chuck, my grandson, by the fireplace. The day before, he had driven his sister and me to the mountains for Thanksgiving. We stopped to have lunch in a small mountain town.

Our waitress approached with a bright smile and enthusiastic recommendations. "If you want banana pudding for dessert, you better order it now. The wait staff ate most of it for breakfast." She was beautiful and enchanting.

On her left shoulder was a large, colorful tattoo that went all the way down to her elbow. On the forearm, writing stretched to her wrist.

When we were back on the road, I mentioned that I found it difficult to understand how a girl so put together would want to have that large tattoo on her arm. It must have been clear to both grandchildren that what I was really saying was, "Don't get a tattoo." We got distracted by another topic and nothing more was said on the ride up.

Later, as we sat by the crackling fire, I again brought it up. I said, "Help me understand how tattoos have become so prevalent. What is going on in the minds of young people to want them? What is it that they say?"

"I knew we were going to have this conversation as soon as that waitress came to our table," said grandson Chuck. "She was right about one thing, the banana pudding was out of sight."

"I agree with that," I said. "But don't change the subject. What's with the tattoos? To me they seem distracting and permanent."

My grandson paused. "Grampy, I'm not sure I'm the one to explain it, but here goes. My favorite teacher, he teaches history. He's also my baseball coach. He has a tattoo on his left arm. He doesn't try to hide it. He will wear short-sleeved shirts and it is easy to see. One day at practice he told us the story about how he came to get it. It has to do with his father and baseball. He said that his father was his coach in every game he played from Little League to American Legion. They won a national championship along the way. He told us that baseball was everything to him. He was sad at the end of every practice and every game. He would end his talks with the words, "Remember, baseball is life."

"His Dad was dying of cancer. He would spend hours with him watching baseball games. The last words his father said was 'Remember, baseball is life.' Coach told us, 'The reason I am coaching is because of him. I had to have a sacred place to write the lines that were so sacred to him so I wrote it in a place that would always be near me, my pitching arm. That's why I have this tattoo.'

"I think that is a pretty cool story, tattoo and all. So one answer for why people get tattoos is to commemorate an important time in their lives or, like Coach, to remember a person who meant a lot to them."

"If I croak, don't get a tattoo," I said.

Chuck shook his head. "I probably won't but no guarantees. It also has become a fad, almost a fashion statement, only permanent. What were the fads when you were in high school?"

I thought for a moment. "A tad less reckless. Believe it or not it was long hair. The Beatles showed up and soon everyone let their hair grow. Parents went nuts. You would have thought civilization itself was on the brink. The fact that one short haircut wiped out the rebellion seemed to be lost on them. With tattoos, momentary, impulsive enthusiasms are permanent. Believe me when I say I would not want symbols of my thoughts and actions as a teenager etched forever anywhere on my body."

My grandson paused again. "You know, Grampy, how Nana always rolls her eyes when you ask waiters and waitresses about themselves. When you say, 'Where are you from?' Or 'Tell us about yourself.'

"It drives her crazy. You told me, in defense of yourself, that the reason you want to know about them is because someone's—everyone's—story has something to teach us. It makes life interesting. I always liked seeing the response from the people you talk to. They like being asked. They like telling their story. If they are young, you ask 'What are your plans?' They really light up when you do that."

"You never backed me up when Nana was around."

"Chalk that up to fear and smarts."

"What does this have to do with tattoos?"

Chuck smiled. "That waitress the other day was smart and funny. She was really pretty. I just knew you would want to know her story, where she was from and her plans for life." He stopped. "But you *didn't*. I think it was the tattoo that turned you off. You missed her story and the connection because you reacted negatively to the tattoo. We have had all kinds of weird waiters and waitresses. They were dressed funky and had crazy hairdos. That never stopped you before. Remember the young guy who waited on us with the hair bun?

"You are still friends with that guy. He always waits on us. I felt sorry for the girl with the tattoo and I felt sorry for you. There was a story there and we missed it."

"You're right. The tattoo put me off."

"Just saying her tattoo may have been like Coach's, a symbol of a loss of something very important to her. Who knows? I don't think that tattoo defines her any more than it defines Coach."

I nodded. "I get it. It's about the person, not the tat. Well said."

Ω

I started this chapter with the definition of relic: *Something that has survived but has lost its original purpose.* The definition terrifies me. The word *remnant* is added on to make it even more intolerable.

If the goal in the *late fragment* is to stay relevant, we must repurpose. The two situations I've presented seem almost trivial on the surface. Too subtle to make the point.

But that IS the point.

The signs that the time has come to actively examine interactions with the world will be whispers and asides, not thunder. Going back to that Thanksgiving conversation when I couldn't get a turn to speak, I am certain there were countless clues to my changing role in the family. I missed them all until I was figuratively hit over the head with a two-by-four.

I keep a journal of what I term "important stuff." This is where I store quotes or ideas that I come across randomly and may want to revisit. I saw the quote, "Be curious, not judgmental," and put it in the journal. It was attributed to Walt Whitman. I came across it recently when I was looking for something else. I thought, "What a curious connection."

What does curiosity have to do with judgment? The conversation I had with my grandson, Chuck, about tattoos provided the shove that finally explained it. He pointed out in his gentle manner that tattoos do not define those who have them. Rather, those who judge them are defined by their contempt. The more issues, thoughts and actions that are criticized and dismissed without curiosity or respectful consideration, the more isolated the person doing the dismissing becomes. Their world becomes small. They eventually lose the knack of connecting or caring. They are hopelessly tied to the past and what seemed to work in "my day."

They are relics.

The antidote to irrelevance is *curiosity*. This is an increasingly complicated world. It shifts every day. If my default mode response is ridicule and rejection—or, worse, contempt—for new, seemingly foreign ideas, my world gets exponentially smaller.

But if I approach odd or incongruous ideas, and people with those ideas, intending to at least understand what they are saying and why they think that way, then my mind and my world is expanding. I don't have to agree. I *do* have to listen, try to understand.

Relevance in the *late fragment* requires that we assume new roles, relinquishing some of the ones we played in previous acts of our lives. One role is that of student.

A student, by definition, doesn't have all the answers. A student is defined by a mindset, not age. He is open to any avenue that can lead him to truth. The role involves seeking knowledge with the hope that it leads to understanding and wisdom. It starts with being curious. Forever.

There is no restriction on the age that one can access understanding and wisdom. The desire to learn and better understand the state of being human doesn't have to wane with age. It is a crucial first step to staying connected to the forces of life.

Curiosity coupled with passion and drive in a young man leads to success. Curiosity coupled with sincerity and tolerance in an old man leads to respect, relevance and love. Being curious about my grandson's take on tattoos and respecting his opinion deepened the connection between generations. It opened a two-way street of learning between us, the young and the old.

As my grandson pointed out, it's not about the tats.

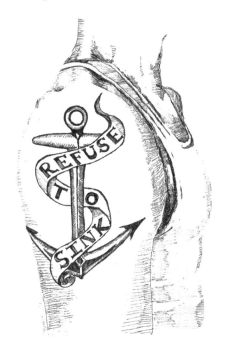

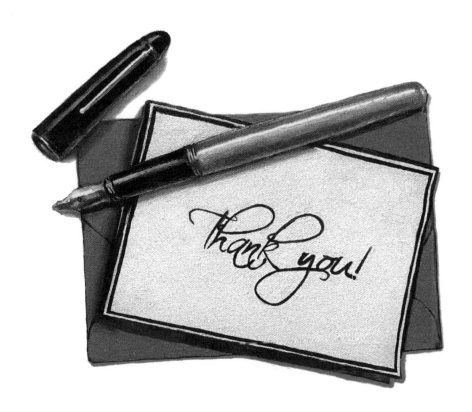

14

Pain and Survival

He who has a why to live can bear almost any how.

Friedrich Nietzsche, "Twilight of the Idols"

As I explained in the introduction, for the past two years I have been consumed with aging lives, lives moving toward the end. Every person I see in my practice, both patient and caregiver, everything I read, every interface and interview with my aging friends is a search for clues and hints that might in some way help me understand this phase of the human journey. I am desperately searching for "AH-HA!" moments that provide insight to offset the crushing pressures that aging imposes. Father Time is a clever and vindictive character. He waits until the exact moment when you think you finally have some of this figured out to throw a curveball which irrevocably changes everything. In the process, he carelessly throws away two qualities that we will need for the future. Trust and hope.

People never seek me out when things are going well. They have no need for what I do. When they do seek me out, the situation is often desperate and always consequential. It places me at the exact moment when life has changed forever. No going back to the familiar, the predictable. I am a part of the unpredictable, scary future. All the fluff, the social agenda, and everything nonessential disappears. We are down to the core, the basics of life. We are now in the survival business.

Survival is more complicated than just the number of days alive. In fact, that is a minor consideration. What "hanging tough" means is keeping as many of the vital elements of lives in play. How can one prevail in the face of staggering adversity? How can relevance, joy, and love stay alive in the phase of life when loss is a constant companion?

Loss has many faces. It can be as mild as arthritic pain from exercise or sports to crippling emotional pain from the loss of a spouse or child. Pain will be there. How we process, negotiate and defy the effects of this pain will determine the quality of the lives that survive.

The point I am trying to make is that how you react to the pain, even seemingly minor throbs, determines not just if you survive but how. Let me explain with two scenarios.

Scenario No. 1

Meet Justin Slayton, nicknamed "Trip." He is a 72-year-old retired chest surgeon from Salem, Va. He had a successful medical career topped off by natural athleticism. Somewhat edgy, but appropriately cocky (he could back it up), he flourished in the world of men. He was a scratch golfer, which he felt excused many of his shortcomings. He was a distant father and strict disciplinarian, even when no discipline was required. His wife was devoted to him in a manner that no longer exists. His adult sons continued to admire him from a distance.

He comes to me with anxiety over memory loss. "I am just not as sharp." The workup reveals Mild Cognitive Impairment, meaning memory loss that doesn't affect everyday life.

His wife adds that she is concerned he has depression. "He is quick to anger and never wants to do anything. He sits all day yelling at the TV."

I am alone with him. My initial impression is that memory loss is not the major deficit. Depression is.

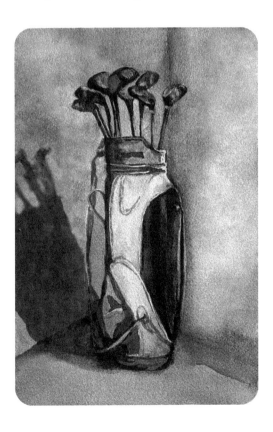

CHE: Trip, Leslie tells me that you have stopped playing golf. Why? Are you injured?

Trip: NO! I am no good anymore. I can't stand shooting in the 80s when I used to shoot in the low 70s.

CHE: You know at our age it's not about the golf but about being out there spending time with your buddies.

Trip: Chuck, save that psychological crap for someone else. You and I have known each other for a long time. You know it won't work on me.

CHE: What about playing with your sons? I know they would enjoy that.

Trip: We don't see much of them. They have their own lives. They don't need to worry about me.

CHE: Leslie says you have lost interest in everything. You don't even follow UVa basketball anymore.

Trip: It just doesn't seem to matter. I'm not interested in much of anything.

CHE: I know you know where I am going with this. My opinion is that you are depressed and have struggled with retirement and the loss of some athletic skills.

Trip: I don't feel sad. How can I be depressed?

CHE: As we age, the evidence of depression is often not sadness. It can be apathy and anhedonia.

Trip: What's anhedonia?

CHE: The loss of pleasure from things you used to love. Your distance from golf would be an example. We also see irritability, anger and the loss of affection for friends and family. Leslie would say you have all of this.

Trip: I'm not sure she is right. I will tell you one thing, I'm not taking any pill to cheer me up and change who I am.

CHE: The antidepressants don't change who you are, they merely return the chemistry in your brain to normal levels. Age often is the culprit in their decline. I want you to let me help you. We can make this better.

Trip: Chuck, thank you. Let me think about it and get back to you.

CHE: Trip, even if you decide not to allow me to treat your depression, you need to get out of the house. You need to reconnect with friends. It is crucial. Rethink this defiance.

Six weeks later

I speak with Leslie on the phone. "Things are even worse," she says. "He has alienated both our sons over money. You had recommended that one have Power of Attorney in light of the early memory loss. He was furious with you and both boys. Memory is declining with more repetitive questions and rapid forgetting. This is so sad. He refuses to come back to see you."

Two years later

I receive a tearful call from Leslie telling me Trip has passed away. She shared that he never softened. He spent two years alone in a chair in front of a TV. Toward the end, he became outraged at everything. Panic set in. He never stopped yelling.

Scenario No. 2

Meet Kristin Kelleher. We'll call her KK. She is a 75-year-old mother of two daughters and grandmother to five granddaughters. She and her husband, John, have been married for 51 years. She stopped working to raise her children.

They would say she was loving and involved but add demanding and suspicious (in a loving way). She has an infectious sense of humor and never misses the funny part. What she was always good at was writing. She loved words and shaping descriptions. She even loved grammar.

The daughters are both success stories and accomplished writers in their own right. "Mom is still our go-to person for guidance, advice and always grammar," they agree.

KK's husband, John, retired last year. Long-delayed travel plans became a reality. You might guess it—she is her own travel agent and not only plans the trips but prepares by reading about every place they travel, in depth.

$$\Omega$$

"I love the whole process." she said in our first conversation. "We really enjoyed several trips early last year. I noticed mild fatigue on the early trips but it became worse later in the year. It was odd because I have always been blessed with energy. I just chalked it all up to being 75.

"Things came apart in Amsterdam. We were booked into the hotel attached to the airport. Even though it was attached, the walk was still more than a half mile. I couldn't make it. We had to stop multiple times because of my shortness of breath. That was the first time I realized something was very wrong.

"It is hard to believe how rapidly my life changed in the span of three days. We returned to Charlotte and I was seen by my primary care physician the next day. One sentence, one simple sentence, changed my life forever. He said, 'Kristin, you have acute leukemia.'

"On the way home, I said the words 'acute leukemia' over and over. I don't know why, I just repeated the words. Two innocuous words.. One means sudden, keen, piercing, sharp. The other cancer of the blood. Maybe I thought repeating the words would make them lose their meaning or lose their sinister power over me.

"I soon realized that those two words would have other words connected to them, like chemotherapy, bone marrow transplant, bone marrow biopsy (OUCH!), transfusion, rejection, death."

I asked her what else she thought and she thought for a moment.

"The first grateful thoughts I had were for having a physician as a husband. It was like having the Amazon Alexa unit at my side to answer any medical questions I had. He also could prepare me for what was coming. Even though he was always truthful about my prognosis, it was calming to have him with me. I would think about the patients who didn't have this medical sage sitting beside them and how frightened and alone they must feel. That may have been the first reason why I never felt sorry for myself. One of my daughters was always with me early on after the transplant. We had a team. I have never felt alone.

"I also knew instinctively that I had to keep my emotions in check. I had to worry about today. Today was going to take all my strength, patience and purpose to survive. I don't let my mind race to places I can't control. This is my life now. I have to make the best of it. Looking back wishing I could have that life back or looking too far forward to not being here serves no purpose.

"The second gift I received, almost miraculously, was a perfect match from a total stranger for the transplant. That person who volunteered to have the biopsy and was a match increased my chances of survival to 80%. I thought of other patients who got sad news, that there was no match or the match was riskier. Things were falling into place. I had to go through the pain. But the odds for success are in my favor."

The bone marrow transplant has been done and KK is at home recovering. She is still controlling her thoughts and keeping her expectations realistic. She never considered herself a victim and never ceased thinking of the plight of others. She has written to every person who reached out to her conveying her sincere gratitude for their thinking of her.

Ω

The two scenarios of Trip and KK share a common theme: Lives irrevocably challenged by health concerns. But they differ in two ways.

The first is in their lives before the challenge. Trip had the impression his favored existence would go on forever without his having to adjust to reality or realizing he had commitments to those who loved him. When the basic components disappeared—the career, the golf—the lack of sustaining factors crushed him. The connection he felt for his friends relied on his expertise at work and golf—not an emotional tie to them as individuals. He could not see or respond to the emotional needs of his wife or sons. Hence he was emotionally bankrupt, emotionally alone.

What would have had to happen to salvage Trip's situation would have been for him to gain the insight that everything in his life that truly mattered was still intact. "I have a devoted family, a lovely wife and sons who at one time wanted to be with me. My memory loss is mild. With my family support, I can make this work."

Sadly, his emotional intelligence fell far short of what was needed. The isolation and defiance accelerated the dementia. The fact that the world had always adapted *to him* tragically prevented him from adapting to new realities in new worlds.

Contrast this outcome with our friend KK. Her life before the bombshell was one of sacrifice. She gave up a career to raise her children and create a loving family. Her dream of traveling the world was upended midstream by the diagnosis. She immediately shifted priorities to adapt to the new realities.

A major component of that shift was controlling her thoughts—the inner dialogue she had with herself. If that inner conversation had resulted in her resentment at the loss of the life she had, she would have pited herself. She might have become a victim. If she allowed her thoughts to project forward to unknowns, fear and anxiety could have taken the place of calm and balance.

But she didn't. Her inner conversation allowed her to show gratitude and grace in the face of dire options. She had always been aware and appreciative of the kindness and generosity of others. The resolve to stay focused on today and its demands permitted her to retain those qualities.

She wrote notes of gratitude to her family and friends, thanking them for their support. She was aware of the gift of a husband who could make medical sense of this outrageous misfortune. She also was aware of the sacrifice of her daughters and of the bone marrow donor, who was an unsuspecting, unsung hero. A lifetime of awareness of others resulted in her receiving affection to ward off despair and loneliness, all the while modeling how to deal with adversity for her children and grandchildren.

This approach allowed her to combat leukemia while Trip couldn't summon the grit to shoot golf scores in the 80s.

These are two rather striking examples which prove the fact that controlling your thoughts allow you to control your actions and hence, control your destiny.

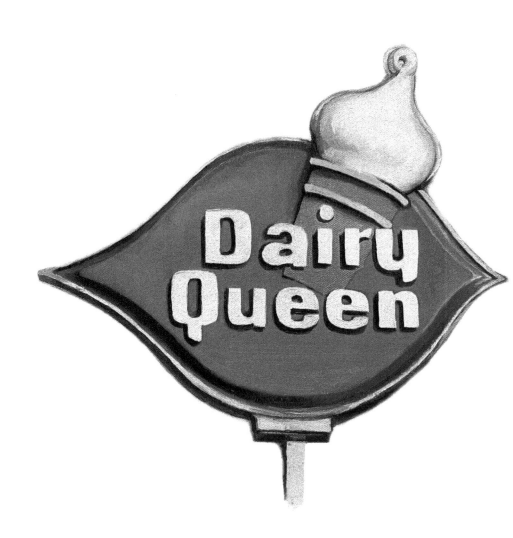

15
So Much Depends On Lunch

Do anything, but let it produce joy.

Walt Whitman

Let me tell you a love story. It involves Alex Jackson and his wife, Norma Berkeley. They have been married 64 years. Alex is 85 years old. Norma is a year older. They live in a retirement community here in Charlotte. Both of them have lived in Charlotte their entire lives.

Alex has been a phenomenon from an early age. He was valedictorian of his high school class and in his class at Princeton. He joined the Marines rather than being drafted, spending two years on active duty just before Vietnam. Following discharge from the service, he turned down scholarships to Harvard and Yale law schools to "come home" to Chapel Hill. It was always odd that Alex was never described as brilliant or even smart. What was said was "He's the kindest person on the planet."

Norma was in the same high school class as Alex but they didn't date until they both wound up in Chapel Hill. She received a Master's degree in English. He studied law. After graduation, they returned home. Norma taught English in the public schools. Alex joined a law firm in Charlotte. They adopted one child, a daughter, Nicole. As you might guess, Alex had a stellar career as a corporate lawyer, sought out for his common sense and insight. Norma was equally successful in her 45 years of teaching. They both worked into their mid 70s.

Retirement was seamless. It gave them more time together doing what they pleased. They traveled the world and enjoyed family and friends. A lifetime passed by. Seven years ago, they moved into a retirement center at the same time as three close couple friends. Initially, they were in a cottage, but three years ago they relocated to the main building in deference to declining mobility.

About the time they made that switch, Alex was involved in an auto accident. While entering on to a busy street past a blind curve, he was hit by an oncoming car. The damage done to both cars was nothing compared to the damage done to Alex's confidence. "I never saw it coming," he explains. Instead of blaming the speed of the other car, he took full responsibility and sadly never drove again. Norma always drove. He sat vigilantly in the passenger seat. The thought that he might hurt someone guaranteed that he was always nervous driving anywhere. They never drove at night and drove only in familiar surroundings.

I will let Alex explain why they came to see me.

AJ: Chuck, I am slowly going downhill with my memory. I struggle with names in the dining room, literally trying to remember the names of people I have known all my life. Norma is amazing with names and covers for me. I have sleep apnea but I no longer am able to follow all the steps in how to use the CPAP. I have quit trying. I know you say that names and technology don't matter, but they matter to me. I know I am slipping and see an uncertain future. Take reading for example.

Norma and I have never watched TV except for sports. We are both readers. Norma is an English teacher. We often will read the same book, sometimes reading to one another. In a new book, I have trouble remembering the storyline from one day to the next. Because of this, we started watching "Masterpiece Theater" on PBS. I need subtitles to understand what they are saying. Even then I lose the plot line.

CHE: So do I.

AJ: I am asking repetitive questions and short-term memory is going.

I meet with Norma alone. She confirms what Alex has shared. She adds, "He always apologizes when he asks me to repeat something. I know it is killing him but it doesn't bother me. At our age, I think we are holding our own."

We do our thing. A careful history, physical exam, neuropsychiatric testing (MOCA in this setting), MRI and full set of labs. His blood pressure is marginally high at 155/88. The MRI shows what are called "white matter changes" slightly more prominent than expected even for him at age 86. White matter changes are historically linked to cardiovascular changes in the brain. The lab is normal. The MOCA score is 26/30 with the only deficits being three losses on ST memory and the date.

For someone at his intelligence level, I feel there is a problem, albeit minor. I explain that this is Mild Cognitive Impairment (MCI). It is defined as mild memory loss that doesn't interfere with everyday life. It is called "amnestic" because at this point it only affects short-term memory. There is no depression. No medication is needed.

Parting advice is simply reassurance.

CHE: Alex, 90% of your life is working in an enviable fashion. We are not going to let the 10% that isn't undermine our happiness. At 85 and 86 years of age, you both are still on the honor roll.

Three-month follow-up. They are together.

CHE: I am happy to report your blood pressure is now acceptable at 138/82. High blood pressure drives memory loss. This positive response will help keep you from declining. I like to know what your routines are. What is going on at your house when things are working? On any given morning when you all wake up and say, 'This is going to be a great day because of this,' what is THIS?

Norma: We are slaves to routine. We get up at the same time every morning, 7:30. We have the same breakfast every day, orange juice, English muffin, red pepper jelly and coffee.

AJ: The English muffin is the crowning achievement of Western civilization.

CHE: I agree.

Norma: If we have family obligations, they would dominate but that is rare. After breakfast, we sit down and plan where we are going for lunch. We eat one major meal a day, always at lunch. It may seem trivial, but we consider it the secret sauce to happiness on a given day.

CHE: I love this. Where do you go?

AJ: Depends on the weather. We have about five go-to places. We rotate depending on different factors. It is a complex and nuanced decision.

CHE: How does the weather come in?

AJ: If it is raining, we can't go to one of them.

CHE: What are the five?

AJ: Phil's Deli, Shake Shack, Chick-fil-A, BrickTop's and Dairy Queen. Each place has a different vibe, not only because of the food but mostly from the different people we encounter there. For instance, BrickTop's is a reservation place. We love some of the dishes but the clientele is affluent and predictable. We like to sit at a vantage point and watch the world go by. There is no place to do that there. We love characters and characters don't hang out at BrickTop's.

CHE: What is your bottom line favorite?

Norma: Dairy Queen, by far.

AJ: No question, Dairy Queen.

CHE: Why?

AJ: First, the food is great. We always split everything. We get a footlong and split it. We have to negotiate the Blizzards.[1] I think the Butterfinger is the bomb but Norma tries to hold out for Heath Bar. But the real reason is the vantage point. There's a park bench next to the outdoor tables. We can see everyone and everything from there. Everyone is equal at Dairy Queen. You wait in line outside, no VIP tables or favored guests. If it's raining, everybody gets wet.

Norma: It is America, waiting in line. It is near the courthouse. Alex recognizes the lawyers standing next to the judge. Right behind them is the defendant with an ankle surveillance device on his ankle. There is something about the line that makes the whole scene authentic. It is just fun to watch.

AJ: There is an indoor/outdoor nursery close by. After we finish, we walk through and see all the orchids. We have to limit how many we buy.

Norma: We love lunch.

Ω

Why is this story important? Why a whole chapter on two people going to lunch? I think you know the answer.

For starters, it's not about lunch. It's about *love*. Why do you think they were able to deal with his memory loss so effectively?

Here is a man who could always rely on one thing in life. It never let him down. His intellect. He was not just smart but a wunderkind.

He is aware that this gift is slowly being taken away. He has lost the ability to follow plot lines and to read for content. However, his saving grace is the devotion from his wife that trumps the memory loss. The apologies for asking repetitive questions are met with affirmation and love. They are a formidable team asking no quarter for the subtle chinks in the armor brought on by their shared longevity.

Anticipation is the human capacity to look forward to, expect, envision the future. It has a positive connotation and is linked to hope and promise. In slang, it is to be "on to something." The something can be anything. It may be lunch, a walk, a big game, bridge, gardening, or an encounter with a person you love. It doesn't matter what, as long as it provides even one skip in a long line of heartbeats.

I would give anything to say that the rituals for Alex and Norma are still in play. Sadly, they are not. Alex survived the first of two strokes and returned close to baseline. The second stroke closed the book—suddenly, thankfully. Norma moved into assisted living immediately. She lost contact with reality without him and declined rapidly.

I have been to the Dairy Queen and sat on the bench where they shared the footlong, the Blizzard and the search for characters. I'm not saying in the grand scheme that this was all that important. No…wait. I'm saying it *is* all that important. It borders on crucial.

In the *late fragment*, our day-to-day routine might not have as big an impact as our actions during our careers. But these rituals are a huge reason that joy and delight are attainable no matter how long we live. They might not involve a major business success. But lunch *is*, after all, lunch and will always be important in its own way. After all, life's huge business deals never come with a Blizzard. Just saying.

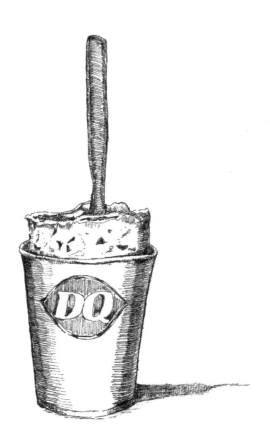

16

Inner Voices

Thoughts become perception, perception becomes
reality. Alter your thoughts, alter your reality.

William James

In each of us, there is an internal conversation that we carry on with ourselves. It is a perpetual back and forth that begins around age two and stops with our last breath. This dialogue is in words, the same words we use to communicate with those in the outside world.[1]

This inner conversation is an instant indication of our attachment to the reality unfolding in front of us. They control our reaction to that reality. The choice of a certain word in this private chat will determine our response to every situation throughout our lives.

The source of the power of this choice of words is in its connection to our authentic selves. We may verbalize to others a different view. But the words in our brain are concretely who we are. In any situation, this inner conversation will control whether we are calm or anxious, positive or negative, or even cowardly or brave. The influence, power, and depth that this internal selection of words has on our thoughts and actions is immeasurable.

The science needed to better understand how all this works has been slow in coming and imprecise. One reason is that researchers are limited in their approaches to the internal conversation of an individual because it depends on that individual sharing their thoughts and describing them precisely.

We do know that the speed of the internal conversation is 10 times faster than when we are speaking to others. This would make the inner pace of words at 4,000 words per minute. These words or sentence fragments instantaneously secure our thoughts and limit the options available to us. It is as if our actions in real time have been predetermined by words created to explain the significance of past, not current events. This whole process—the speed, control and consequences—is breathtaking in its power and pervasiveness.

All our life is but a mass of small habits—
practical, emotional, intellectual and spiritual—
that bear us irresistibly toward our destiny.

William James

I know I am hitting William James hard here. But it is impossible to take on this subject of internal dialogue without him. He is the father of American psychology and early on wrote about many aspects of the human experience that have survived unscathed from both academia and pop culture. The quote above is witness to his genius. He realized that life is an accumulation of experiences that add to the vocabulary of our inner thoughts. That vocabulary always determines what we think, what we say, and what we do—what he refers to as our destiny.

I am going to briefly bring back two characters from previous chapters to illustrate what I mean.

In the chapter, "The Sin of Pride," we struggled along with Randal, the retired lawyer who lost his wife of 56 years to pancreatic cancer. He presented to the clinic with an abnormal grief reaction characterized by depression. The sadness and confusion were triggered by regret, resulting in suicidal thoughts.

In my initial plan for him, I explained that I was going to start him on medication to help with anxiety, obsessions and depression. I added that no medication was up to this task without his controlling the conversation he has with himself.

The loneliness had allowed the internal conversation to be dominated by the words *regret, pride, lonesome, pain* and *stop*. The depression prevented any positive anticipation for the future by not allowing the words *forgive, obligation, promise, love, worthy, happy* and *hope*.

His life going forward would hinge on actions determined by the words he chose to use. The simple strategy of reintroducing him to himself and bringing loved ones back into play slowly changed the inner vocabulary. I need to FORGIVE myself. I have OBLIGATIONS to those I love. I have PROMISES to keep to those departed. I am WORTHY of this LOVE. I now have HOPE that the future holds HAPPINESS for me.

This process of actively controlling the words we speak to ourselves is more effective than any medication. It has the power to change lives.

The second person I want to revisit is KK. She is the 75-year-old mother/grandmother who was diagnosed with acute leukemia. The sudden, devastating diagnosis was a perfect setting for *denial, pity, retrospect* and *anger*. She refused to allow those words to take hold. The words she chose were *now, grateful, fortunate* and *please*.

She says this is my life NOW. No wishful looking back mourning the loss of what was. I am GRATEFUL for my husband who is able to guide and support me and for my family, which is at my side. I am FORTUNATE to have a perfect match from a total stranger. And lastly, PLEASE, Lord, give me the strength to live up to the pain and fears that are in my immediate future. The words transformed into actions on every count. An added effect is the example to her children and grandchildren on how to deal with the vicissitudes of life that are certain and ahead.

These are two examples of how carefully selecting the words with our inner voice provides options for overcoming uncertainties. It is the bedrock of resilience and survival.

There is a caveat here. One cannot wait until the lightning has struck to choose the appropriate word for the occasion. Each interaction with reality has the potential to add new words to the working vocabulary. If the world is approached with the respect and reverence it deserves, each encounter brings a new and unique perspective. This process adds words or increases the scope and meaning of the words we already possess. Over a lifetime, this results in an exponential increase in understanding this human journey. It is called wisdom.

The English language is the perfect vehicle for the accumulation of words and actions needed for all seasons. In the Oxford English Dictionary, there are 500,000 words.[2] The Germans have 185,000 words in their dictionary. The French have fewer than 100,000. English provides us with an abundance of words which allow us to interact with others and respond to an abundance of situations—some good, some not.

Each situation we encounter evokes a response from our inner vocabulary. The words we select determine our attitude toward the reality that is unfolding. They put a spin on everything. That spin is either positive or negative.

Let me show you what I mean.

A situation can be…
*   tragic
*   abhorrent
*   abusive
*   unsavory
*   unpleasant
*   unacceptable

Or a situation can be…
*   marginal
*   tolerable
*   so-so
*   acceptable
*   preferable
*   enviable
*   joyful
*   ideal
*   sublime
*   perfect

There is a great distance between "tragic" and "perfect." You get the idea. When your senses confront a situation or event, they transmit that information to your brain. The brain triages as many factors about this situation as possible, instantaneously. That evaluation, those factors, are conveyed to the consciousness in words.

The slant we take away from this interface with reality is biased by our life experiences—the patterns and habits resulting from similar past interfaces with the external world. Our history has created a lexicon, a personal dictionary, that stores every experience in our lives. These words are available to guide us in familiar surroundings. But the bias they are tethered to may not be appropriate in new circumstances.

If one is not inclined to be curious or inquisitive about unfolding events, then new words that are indispensable to understanding our personal narratives are suppressed. They never come into play. We are hopelessly trapped in our own past.

The anxiety related to advancing age exaggerates this tendency to use words that no longer explain reality. The relevance we long for throughout our lives depends on the creation of new words in our inner voice. Words that reflect a fascination with this evolving world and the humans in it.

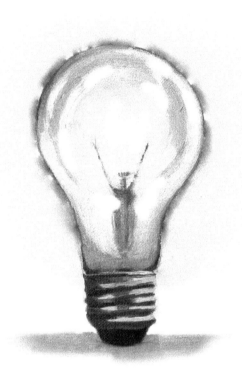

17

Just Between Us

When two people relate to each other authentically and
humanly, God is the electricity that surges between them.

Martin Buber

I recently read the book *Sapiens: A Brief History of Humankind* by
Yuval Noah Harari.[1] It is an enlightened, exhaustive dive into the
sole-surviving species of humans, *Homo Sapiens* (Wise Men). Early
in the book, he attempts to answer the crucial question in evolution:
Why did *our* species, homo sapiens, survive over the other human
species that existed with them? He covers several theories and the
evidence for each, then opts for one called the "replacement" theory.
This explanation requires a mutation that occurred 70,000 years ago,
resulting in a profound survival advantage.

What was that advantage? More important, why would I start
this chapter in a book on aging lives with *that* question? How possibly
could they be connected? If they *are* connected, what difference could
it make to an aging individual in the 2020s?

This survival advantage was our *ability to communicate with each
other.* The mutation was the first step in the development of language

that was adaptable to reality. It involved sharing observations, problems, ideas, solutions, and gossip about others. Through the mutated DNA, we are hardwired for human interaction and communication. We are genetically programmed to rely on one another, share our fears and dreams with one another, care for one another. When we are isolated or reclusive, we give up our genetic inheritance that is crucial to our happiness and feelings of security and well-being.

This may be the most important chapter in the book. It, along with "So Much Depends On Lunch," speaks directly to joy and purpose every day. It is undeniable that one cannot have a happy month, year, or decade without a predominance of happy days. The truth is that aging, coupled with distance from other humans, has the potential to rob us every day of the feelings of being whole and relevant. We need each other to feel complete.

Age and the travails of a lifetime enhance social anxiety. This is a recipe for loneliness, depression and despair. The question I asked Randal on our first visit was, "How many days a week do you go without seeing another human being?" When he responded, "Does waving at my neighbor count?" the answer was "NO!" He admitted to five days. This was a red flag for lurking troubles.

Human interaction plays an indispensable role in keeping minds sharp and lives worth living. The simple act of listening to another person talk activates chemicals in our brain that force us to react to what is being said. There are different chemicals produced when we like what we hear as opposed to when we disagree. We need no further proof that this process exists and is controlling of our emotion than when a series of spoken words incite a violent rage.

Just as important—perhaps *more* important—is being listened to and understood. This verbal back and forth are the source of value in lives. These interfaces are the conduits through which self-worth, compassion, and love are conveyed to other humans. One begins to sense the impact and importance of this interplay when saying to or hearing from another person the words, "I love you."

The presence of humans and the vocabulary of that presence is essential to everything that follows in our lives. It is not the only element. But without it, the other factors have difficulty replacing it. Let's take a look at the beginnings of human interaction that occur within families and spread out from there.

> There is no vocabulary
> For love within a family, love that's lived in
> But not looked at, love within the light of which
> All else is seen, the love within which
> All other love finds speech.
> This love is silent.
>
> T.S. Eliot
> "The Elder Statesman"

The first, and for most of us, most important interactions with other humans is within families. As Eliot states, it is love that is "lived in." Each family has its own dynamic—its unique manner in which members interact, show concern for one another, love each other. For those born into a certain family, this unique manner is all they know. It is only later, from a distance as adults, that the positives and negatives are examined and their impacts weighed.

The effect of this family dynamic has lifelong, profound consequences. If a family is loving and demonstrative in that love, the child learns how to give and receive affection. If the family is reserved and uncomfortable with displays of affection, the child may always be uncomfortable with emotional demonstrations. The point is that our initial lessons in human interaction are inside our families. Those basic lessons affect every encounter and relationship we have throughout our lives.

The chemistry between family members, their commitment to each other and to the family in general, is complicated. There is an unreal expectation that families are the source of unconditional love and eternal support throughout one's life. The majority of families fall short of that ideal on some level. The emotional reaction to that shortfall, because of societal expectation, is always out of proportion and often hurtful.

Each of us has an idea of how a family should work from our own experience with our parents, siblings and relatives. We are also intensely interested in how other families work. "Tell me about your family" is a common starting point for new relationships. Psychotherapy usually starts with the same statement.

My learning curve on this subject rose dramatically when I began caring for patients with memory loss. The diagnosis of dementia in a parent, brother, or sister puts crushing pressures on families. The societal stigma and alarming reality of the prognosis creates fault lines.

My goal is to keep the patient calm, safe, clean and loved throughout the illness. I can only do that by working with the family as the primary caregivers. The more effective those caring for the patient are, the better chance I have of achieving my goals. Those fault lines come into play immediately and are present long after the patient is gone.

Let me show you what this looks like in action.

Ω

Henry Blake is a 66-year-old caregiver for his 94-year-old mother, Clara. He makes an appointment to see us, saying, "I need help with my mother."

They arrive together. She walks in the clinic without assistance.

The three of us sit down for a conversation.

Henry: Dr. Edwards, let me give you some necessary background. My mother has been living in our family home in High Point, N.C., since my dad died more than 30 years ago. She is fiercely independent. She will allow no caregivers to come in to help. Two months ago, she fell in the bathroom, fracturing her hip. She underwent surgery and just finished a month of rehab. I arranged for the rehab to be here in Charlotte. I felt she was no longer able to live independently. That time has run out. She is not happy.

CHE (to Clara): First, let me tell you how impressed I am with your recovery from the fracture. You seem to have sailed through the operation and rehab at 93. You are amazing. You do have to admit Charlotte is a much nicer town than High Point.

Clara: I know you are baiting me, but I will admit no such thing. (She says this with a smile.) Dr. Edwards, you are aware my son has me locked up in a prison. That retirement home.

Henry: It is not a prison. You make it a prison by not getting out of your room. You need to meet people and participate in all the stuff we are paying for.

Clara: I am 93 years old. I have met all the people I want to meet in this life.

CHE: Are you still getting physical therapy for your balance and gait so you don't fall again?

Clara: I am. They insist I use a walker. I don't feel I need it. I have fallen once in 93 years. I am not a cripple. One fall and I give up my life. My cats, my house, everything. I don't think either of you would tolerate this. I know Henry wouldn't.

Henry: You see what I am up against. She refuses to act rationally. I just don't want her to fall.

We spend 20 minutes learning her history and listening to her side of the story. She is repetitive but her social skills are intact. We separate. I am alone with Henry.

Henry: Dr. Edwards, you can see my problem. She either is refusing to cooperate, which would be typical, or she is now incapable of it. Either one is tough on me. I want her to be happy, but there are limits to how understanding I can be.

CHE: Are there times when your visits work, when you feel like you are getting through? For 93, she is pretty sharp. She can't live alone but dementia is not a major issue here.

Henry: Our visits follow a pattern. She is glad to see me. It is odd. She has trouble hearing everyone else but has no trouble following everything I say, even in a normal voice. We will have a nice conversation about the day.

Predictably, after a short interlude, obsessions take over. She misses her cats and tries to make the case that she can return home to High Point. She negotiates that she will allow help to come in if I sign off on the return. To be fair, she is actually pretty reasonable with all that. I think she knows that in many ways she is better off here, certainly less anxious. She doesn't want to admit it, at least not to me.

CHE: Sounds OK up to now.

Henry: Then it goes off course. She starts in on what a wonderful person my father was and what a wonderful husband and dad he turned out to be. None of that is true. He was a drunk, simple fact. Eventually he drank himself to death. My life up until the day I left for college was dominated by alcohol, anger and shame. She never talks about the embarrassment he caused all of us. He would show up at games drunk. Even as a young boy, I refused to go into a restaurant with him.

CHE: Can't you let those false memories of hers go by, just to keep the peace?

Henry: I can't. To be honest, I haven't tried. Look, I left home at 17 to go to Chapel Hill. I never returned home for any length of time afterward. I swore that I would never live the lie that things were OK. They weren't. He doesn't deserve that rewriting of history. I cannot allow her to create this alternate reality. The truth matters, and it especially matters to me in this setting.

CHE: Weren't all of you hurt by his drinking? How did she cope with it?

Henry: She couldn't stand up to him. She tried to hide it as best she could. When I was around 8 or 9, she would have me sneak in his study and bring the liquor bottles out so she could add water. She hoped that by doing that, it wouldn't get too bad. She made a decision early on that she was going to stick it out and she did. If pressed, she would say she did it for me and my sister.

I love my mother. While he was alive, she shared the torment with us. I want to know why she insists on forgetting what he was really like. I just can't go where she wants me to. Too many demons.

CHE: What do you do?

Henry: I tell her to stop. Her false memories insult us both. I won't hear them.

CHE: What does she do?

Henry: She says the same thing every time. She says, "You know his father was the same way. They shared a tragic flaw." She then tells me the same story about a time on vacation in Blowing Rock that one night, late, they danced alone in the parking lot to the radio. Maybe it's true, maybe not. But I never heard that story before. It's the same thing every time. I leave feeling bad for her and for my distance from her. I just can't share any good memories of him. I don't have any. I would be the biggest phony if I let all this go by.

CHE: I can't believe you don't have any good memories of your dad. I know you have something.

Henry: It's strange that you should mention this. The other day two distinct memories came into my brain. I hadn't thought of either one in years. The first was at a picnic when I was 11. All my friends and their families were there. We were playing softball. I was playing right field. My dad was playing center. He was a good athlete early in his life. One of the fathers hit a line drive between my dad and me. It was hit hard. I knew it would be a home run. My dad caught it on the dead run with his back to home plate. No one could believe it. It was Willie Mays-like. It was the one time I can remember I was proud of him in the face of other people.

The second was one Saturday morning when he took me to the furniture store to show me something he had just bought. He was proud of it and wanted me to see it. It was a computer that tracked every piece of furniture in the store and automatically reordered stuff that was selling out. He sat down and played the computer like a piano. He took me to lunch, just the two of us. He got excited about the future of computers. I remember he said that soon every business and possibly every home would have one. He wanted me to know that.

CHE: Your company is involved with computers, right?

Henry: Yes, mostly software. I can see where you're going. I hope you understand that one catch and one lunch is a sad counterweight to a lifetime of disappointment.

CHE: I get it. But it's nice to have something. Back to your mom. What would it take to make this special time in both your lives to work?

Henry: That's why I am here. So far it's not even close to where we need to be.

CHE: First, you deserve credit for making good decisions on her behalf. The nuts and bolts are all in place. You are doing everything right on the checklist. But long-established demons are undermining the closeness and understanding you both long for. You both have been damaged emotionally by the tragic effect of your dad's drinking. Both your brains are playing tricks on you.

Henry: Tricks? I know what happened.

CHE: Let me explain. Your mother refuses to go near the tormented memories she has regarding your dad. If she gets near them, anxiety takes over. She then diverts to thoughts that counter that uneasiness. This ritual has allowed her peace and space from the pain for 30 years. When she goes near those suppressed agonies, the calm and pleasantness disappear. The trick the brain plays is creating the illusion that much of the pain didn't happen. Therefore it accentuates the good times even if they are sparse. Dancing with him in the parking lot in Blowing Rock is one of those tricks. It may have happened. Maybe not. But it is her reality and allows her memories of when things worked and she was happy.

You, on the other hand, are doing the exact opposite. The anger you have for your dad is a daily factor in your life. The trick your brain plays on you is even more sinister. Your anxiety and uneasiness with life is at a low point when your rage at him is present. When you are asked or forced to move away from the anger, anxiety explodes. You have already referred to it once, "I said I would never accept the lie that it didn't happen."

This puts you in the presence of anger too often. Anger has a way of spilling over into places it doesn't belong. It makes matters worse. Even with your impressive successes, that feeling never leaves. It's as if you insist that if I am not edgy or outright angry then I am not being true to myself. It is always right there under the surface. But you don't get the connection. You get angry easily over seemingly trivial things. I'll bet you later say to yourself, "Why did I get mad over that? It wasn't even remotely important."

Henry: That happens all the time. I can blow up over silly stuff. It has been my Achilles' heel.

CHE: Instead of avoiding it like your mother, you have done the opposite. You have placed it at the center of who you are and what you see. You mistakenly have the idea that if I don't keep these resentments alive, I will condone what happened. That obsession is preventing you from seeing your mom's predicament in a soft light.

    She is 93. I want you to come to grips with this before we lose her and lose the opportunity to have you come to peace with it. Regret is something we have the option to avoid.

Henry: Aren't you my mother's doctor? I don't have any recollection of making an appointment for myself. (Delivered with a smile).

CHE: I can't help your mom unless I help you. All I'm trying to do is make you aware of factors that prevent you from seeing your mom and making this all work. The image I have is of you two plotting together to water down your dad's whiskey. I want that team back.

Henry: Dr. Edwards, I think I get some of this. I do appreciate where you're coming from. This is a lot for me to handle.

CHE: I am going to check some labs and image her brain with a quick CT. She is 93. She does not need a complex workup. We reconvene in one week.

You have one task in that week. I would usually say to step back and rethink your role. But stepping away from it is not the answer. I want you to step toward her. See her. What is unresolved between you and your dad has to be set aside. It probably never had a right to be placed between mother and son. But if it did, the reason for it is gone. What she needs at this point is affirmation.

She needs to hear that she was a good mother. She needs to hear that in a way that makes up for some of the pain you both endured. It is that simple. See you in one week.

One week later. I am alone with Henry.

CHE: Tell me where you are. I know this week has been tough.

Henry: Tough would be an understatement. Torture would be close, persecution even closer. I won't lie to you. There was a part of me that was angry over the things you said. I questioned whether you had the authority to wade in so personally on me. That resentment lasted one day.

Two things you said that I couldn't get off my mind. The first was that I was allowing the rage at my father to blind me from seeing my mother. When she would say "He was a good husband or father" and my blood would boil. I was thinking, "You silly old woman, how can you forget how much he hurt you and me! Don't you get it?"

Maybe I ran out of anger. I finally saw her without the rage at him. I realized that I want her happy. I also came to the realization that I am the only one on any level who could make that happen.

What was especially painful was the fact that she needed to hear the words you said and I have been unwilling to say them. I have to do this on my terms. But I get it.

You might not be aware but I do have positive qualities. One of them is negotiation. I thought, "If I wanted to turn this around, where would I start?"

It was as if I was slapped across the face with the answer. THE CATS!! I called the facility and learned they have a corridor that allowed pets. I called my sister and asked her to bring the cats to our house. The next day, I arranged for lunch with my mother. During that lunch, all her belongings were transferred to her new room on the "pet corridor."

My wife brought the cats to the new room and mom was reunited with them. I negotiated a harsh truce. Any talk of returning to High Point would involve the disappearance of the cats. We also are trying to leverage this into some physical therapy. It's a start. She was ecstatic.

CHE: Wow. I am impressed.

Henry: The second thing you said was the hardest to get my arms around. It was when you connected my resentment with everything about my father with my quick temper. That hit me hard. The reality played out in painful waves of recognition. It started with, "Yes I'm outraged by what happened to me. I am justified by my anger at it." It ended with the realization that I had allowed the early misfortune in my life to follow me and often control me. I actually hid behind it. It allowed me to always set the rules for myself. The No. 1 rule has been, "If I can't control it, I don't play." I've been hurt enough in this lifetime. Losing control has the potential for pain.

CHE: You have been on to this for a while. It didn't start with our talk.

Henry: You are right. I've been aware for a long time that my reaction to things wasn't working. I am always on defense. What came out of our discussion over mom was the barrier that the anger created. Connecting the rage to the feeling that I have gotten a bad deal in life was what opened my eyes. As long as I stay pissed off, I'm tethered to the pain I experienced as a child. I can't get past it. We'll see how this goes.

CHE: These are huge steps. My goal was simply to have you enjoy seeing your mom at 93 dancing in the parking lot in Blowing Rock. I love seeing the team back in action.

She lived four more years. Toward the end, she was blind and deaf. The one person who was allowed into her private world was her son, Henry. Everyone else had to yell. He could speak softly and connect effortlessly. The emotional truce became a special haven for both mother and son. Old wounds healed. Regrets died.

$$\Omega$$

The Blakes' story reveals how important coming to resolutions in families is for multiple generations. Awareness and forgiveness in the *late fragment* can lead to peace at the end for the departing, and a fortifying confidence for those left behind.

All happy families are alike—each unhappy family is unhappy in their own way.

— Tolstoy —

First lines of *Anna Karenina*

When Families Don't Work, What Then?

A nameless woman stops me in the parking lot following a talk I have just given. She apologizes for stopping me, saying, "I have one question to ask but was too shy to ask in front of all those people."

CHE: Shoot.

Lady: I am 75 years old and live alone in a single- family house on Bywood Lane here in Charlotte. I have been divorced from my husband now for more than 15 years. I have two children, an older daughter who lives in Oregon and a son who lives here. For different reasons, I am estranged from them both. I have made multiple attempts to reconcile, forgive and be forgiven. All have failed. When you spoke on how important interactions with families are, it struck a sensitive chord. My question is "What do I do now? I feel alone and helpless."

CHE: Tell me your name.

Lady: My name is Sylvia Patton. Dr. Edwards, I feel I have been treated unfairly. I was a good mother and wife. I don't deserve this isolation.

CHE: Sylvia, it's nice to meet you. I agree that no one deserves isolation.

Sylvia: I apologize for dumping my personal problems on you. I have nowhere else to turn. When I saw you, I impulsively said, "This is my chance," so I took it.

CHE: This is fine. You asked me a specific question. What can one do when family fails an individual? It seems that you have completed Step No. 1, trying to make it work through contact, understanding and forgiveness. Reconciliation is always the preferred option. But there are times when all avenues to harmony are blocked.

My first option is always met with exasperation. It's always keep trying to mend fences with family. The stakes are too high to let hurt feelings and exasperation prevent potential harmony or even a negotiated truce.

Sylvia: I have done all that. What is Option No. 2?

CHE: Option No. 2 is to create a new family. You are related to this new family not by genetics but by awareness, caring and love. These are individuals you want to talk with, listen to, and share experiences.

Seeking out friends of this kind is invaluable even when your "real family" is involved and supportive. The new family can emerge from a number of places in your life. Often, individuals sharing common experiences or challenges seek new friends. This is especially common among our caregivers. Special friends may be recycled old friends with whom you have lost touch. They may be right next door. They may be work colleagues who, like you, have retired and are now alone. It doesn't matter where they come from. What matters is that they are essential in aging lives.

Sylvia: How do you go about this? Right now, I have been hurt so much that I am thinking I don't need any more rejection.

CHE: You are right. The process of connecting to others involves risk. But the rewards are worth the uneasiness. Yes, there are individuals out there who have no need for new avenues of human contact. They are fortunate to have loving families. Children, grandchildren and great-grandchildren hold a special place in their lives. But I have seen the opposite. In the *late fragment,* a decline in mobility and the actual loss of contemporaries can rob a person of caring relationships. Having a friend with whom to share the challenges of aging would be a gift. Better yet, to have a fellow maverick who is willing to conspire with you to trick Father Time and stave off the disrespects of aging would be joyous. Believe me, they are out there in abundance.

Sylvia: On a practical level, how does one go about this? Do I pick up the phone and call someone and say, "My life is really not working out. I need someone to help me. I have chosen you?" I doubt that is going to end up in a good place.

CHE: How you go about this is up to you. These individuals may already be in your life and you have forgotten them. Or they are new to you and need to be discovered. Who, where, and when is your deal.

Sylvia: I got it. I have to be bold to make this work.

CHE: When you begin to connect with new or old friends, be the friend to them that you want them to be to you. Things will fall into place.

Sylvia: Thank you.

I have tried to find Sylvia but have failed. The group I spoke to that day has no record of a Patton on Bywood Lane. I hope that she not only has found a new family but that her old family has resolved its painful differences.

Ω

This scenario is all too common—a woman living alone and feeling abandoned. Forming connections with other humans is essential for happiness in each phase of our lives. The *late fragment* often presents roadblocks to finding such fulfilling relationships. This story and these suggestions are an attempt to make all of us aware of the unique burdens faced by those who live alone. More importantly, I have tried to make individuals suffering from isolation aware that there is hope for them to reconnect with fellow humans. But it requires risk and boldness. I repeat myself for emphasis. The rewards are incalculable.

I actually take issue with Tolstoy. Each happy family is happy in its own way just as each unhappy family is unhappy in its own way. The complexities of life—timing, health, fortune and misfortune—make it so. This is complicated stuff, complicated and fragile. And yet two truisms cut through the *late fragment*:

1. It is hard enough to survive with loved ones close by. Without loved ones in the picture, it is lonely and scary.

2. You will gradually lose individuals you respected and cherished. Death closes some of those relationships. Some are ended by loss of mobility. Others by common interests no longer being in play. Bridge partners must take on new roles if neither are playing bridge. Reactivating these connections through new shared experiences is vital to sustaining human interaction. It might be as simple as enjoying breakfast or going to a baseball game with a friend. Whatever it is, the anticipation and shared experience will make it all worthwhile.

The studies tell us what we know in our hearts. Lives are longer and happier when shared with another.

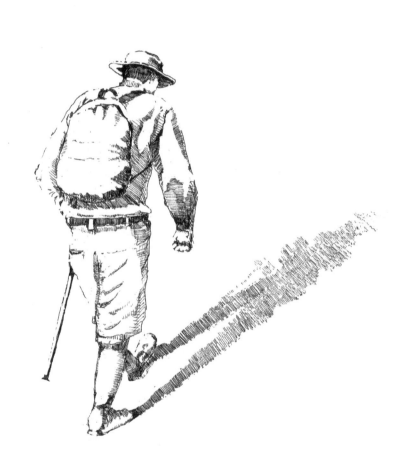

Before I Go

Gratitude bestows reverence allowing us to encounter everyday epiphanies, those transcendent moments of awe that change forever how we experience life and the world.

John Milton

So it comes down to this, a final moment at the end of this odyssey on aging and the human experience. The three years I devoted to writing this book have been life-changing for me on countless levels. The individuals I interviewed, interacted with, watched, and now remember have provided a lesson plan that has reduced fears of the future and reinforced the importance of connections to fellow humans.

Many of the individuals I interviewed and befriended are no longer with us. Their fate has played out. I am comforted by the fact that their struggles and triumphs are preserved in this book. Their counsel will be available when we need it.

The final question that you need to ask is this: After all the searching, listening and talking, is there a takeaway, a final observation expressed by those individuals who survived or even flourished in the *late fragment*? Is there a secret to true success?

The answer is yes. But it is not a secret. John Milton shared it with us in this chapter's opening quote. It is *gratitude*. I saw it over and over. When I asked the question of an older colleague, "What makes all this work?" I knew what was coming. The answer was always "Gratitude." Gratitude has nothing to do with career success, financial security, or social standing. It is plainly dismissive of the trappings of ego. It has little to do with personal triumphs and financial acquisitions.

Sadly, there were many people I interviewed who did not get the "human memo." Their obsession with "What I have achieved?" makes them compete with one another until the end. This keeps them from forming those pure attachments to other humans, and the profound sense of well-being that comes from them.

But those who *did* get it? In expressing gratitude for those pure attachments, what they were conveying was the security and joy derived from being human and being among humans. From being loved and being able to love. This became clear in the stories they told, what they valued, what raised their spirits. They were drinking from a spring that flowed from the depths of this earthly experience. They were calm, fearless, appreciative, reverent. Humility tagged along.

I entitled the last part of the book "Directive." That's the title of a magnificent poem by Robert Frost. In it, he walks us through an abandoned landscape to a hidden spring that he claims drinking from can "make us whole again beyond confusion."

That was my intent for this book from the beginning. I wanted to make us aware of time, how precious it is because of its eventual limit. I wanted to shock us into turning away from the details that no longer matter. I wanted to connect us to the legacy left by those who got it and to see the path set for those of us who will follow.

For me, I have loved our time together.

Endnotes

Introduction

1. Edwards II, Dr. C.H. *Much Abides: A Survival Guide for Aging Lives*. United Writers Press. 2020.

Chapter 1: Age and Culture

1. I cannot recall where or when I read about the Bedouin legend. I also cannot explain why it stuck with me. It may not be true. I have no evidence for that possibility either. However, there is documented evidence that nomadic/tribal communities frequently left their elders in this similar manner:

Lin, J. "Scholar intrigued by how societies treat their elderly." UCLA Center for Near Eastern Studies, *UCLA Today*. 2010, January 7. https://www. International .ucla.edu/cnes/article/113384

Diamond, J.M. (2012) *The world until yesterday: What can we learn from traditional societies?* Viking.

Chapter 2: A Gift Of Time?

1. Arias, E., Tejada-Vera, B., Kochanek, K.D. & Ahmed, F.B. (2022, August) Vital Statistics Rapid Release. National Center for Health Statistics. https//www.cdc.gov/nchs/data/vsrr/vsrr023.pdf

2. Population projections for the United States from 2015 to 2060, by detailed age group. Statistica, Statistica Research Department. (2014, December). https://www.statistica.com/statistics/611644/united-states-population-projection-by-age/

Chapter 3: Even So

1. Carver, R. *A new path to the waterfall: Poems.* Atlantic Monthly Press. 1989.

2. King, S. "Raymond Carver's life and stories." *The New York Times*, 1. (2009, November 19). http://www.nytimes.com/2009/11/22/books/review/King-t.html

3. Bauer, J.(n.d.) Raymond Carver. Poetry Foundation; Poetry Foundation.org/poets/Raymondcarver

Chapter 5: Limits Of Devotion

1. De la Monte, S.M. & Goel, A. "Agent Orange Reviewed: Potential Role in Peripheral Neuropathy and Neurodegeneration." *Journal of Military and Veteran's Health*, 2002, 30(2), 17-26.

2. Martinez, S., Yaffe, K., Li,Y., Byers, A.L. et al. "Agent Orange Exposure and Dementia Diagnosis in U.S. Veterans of the Vietnam Era." *JAMA neurology*, 78(4), 473-477. https://doi.org/10.1001/jamaneurol. 2020.5011

Chapter 6: The Sin Of Pride

1. Pride is considered the most egregious of the seven deadly sins. Also referred to as the cardinal sins, they are Pride, Gluttony, Lust, Envy, Greed, Wrath and Sloth. In a fundamentalist Baptist church, pride is an unforgivable sin. Sands, P. (n.d.). The deadly sin of pride. Baylor University School of Social Work: Family and Community Ministries, 40-49.

Chapter 7: The Science Of Despair

Living Alone

1. Ausubel, J. Older people are more likely to live alone in the U.S. than elsewhere in the world. Pew Research Center; Pew Research Center. https://www.pewresearch.org/short-reads/2020/03/10/older-people-are-more-likely-to-live-alone-in-the-u-s-than-elsewhere-in-the-world/#:~:text=In%20the%20U.S.%2C%2027%25%20of,130%20countries%20and%20territories%20studied.

2. Fung, H.H. Aging in culture. *The Gerontologist*, 2013, 53(3), 369–377. https://doi.org/10.1093/geront/gnt024.

3. Kaplan, D.B. "Older Adults Living Alone." *Merck Manual Professional Version.* 2023, April. Merck. https://www.merckmanuals.com/professional/geriatrics/social-issues-in-older-adults/older-adults-living-alone

4. Molinsky, J. The Number of People Living Alone in Their 80s and 90s is Set to Soar. Housing Perspectives: Research, Trends, and Perspective from the Harvard Joint Center for Housing Studies; Joint Center for Housing Studies of Harvard University (2020, March 10). https://www.jchs.harvard.edu/blog/the-number-of-people-living-alone-in-their-80s-and-90s-is-set-to-soar.

5. Seegert, L. Culture an important factor in 'successful' aging. Covering Health: Monitoring the Pulse of Health Care Journalism; Association of Health Care Journalists. (2013, November 22). https://healthjournalism.org/blog/2013/11/culture-an-important-in-gauging-successful-aging/

Loneliness

6. Delgado-Losada, M.L., Bouhaben, J., Arroyo-Pardo, E., Aparicio, A., & López-Parra, A. M. "Loneliness, Depression, and Genetics in the Elderly: Prognostic Factors of a Worse Health Condition?" *International journal of environmental research and public health.* 2022. 19 (23), 15456. https://doi.org/10.3390/ijerph192315456

7. Lapane, K.L., Lim, E., McPhillips, E., Barooah, A., Yuan, Y., & Dube, C.E. Health effects of loneliness and social isolation in older adults living in congregate long term care settings: A systematic review of quantitative and qualitative evidence. *Archives of gerontology and geriatrics*, 2022, 102, 104728. https://doi.org/10.1016/j.archger.2022.104728.

8. Ong, A.D., Uchino, B.N., & Wethington, E. Loneliness and Health in Older Adults: A Mini-Review and Synthesis. *Gerontology*. 2016. 62(4), 443–449. https://doi.org/10.1159/000441651

9. Stanford SPARQ Department of Psychology. (n.d.). UCLA Loneliness Scale (Version 3). Stanford |SPARQtools; Stanford University. https://sparqtools.org/mobility-measure/ucla-loneliness-scale-version-3/

Depression

10. Cai, H., Jin, Y., Liu, R., Zhang, Q., Su, Z., Ungvari, G. S., Tang, Y. L., Ng, C. H., Li, X. H., & Xiang, Y. T. (2023). Global prevalence of depression in older adults: A systematic review and meta-analysis of epidemiological surveys. *Asian journal of psychiatry*, 80, 103417. https://doi.org/10.1016/j.ajp.2022.103417

11. Depression In Older Adults: More Facts. Mental Health America; Mental Health America. 2023. https://www.mhanational.org/depression-older-adults-more-facts.

12. Oon-arom, A., Wongpakaran, T., Kuntawong, P., & Wongpakaran, N. "Attachment anxiety, depression, and perceived social support: a moderated mediation model of suicide ideation among the elderly." *International psychogeriatrics*, (2021), 33(2), 169–178. https://doi.org/10.1017/S104161022000054X

13. Rodriguez, F. (2019, August 28). How Many Senior Citizens Have Depression? SucessTMS; Success TMS. https://successtms.com/blog/depression-in-the-elderly-statistics#:~:text=Between%201%25%20and%205%25%20of,the%20depression%20rate%20is%2013.5%25.

14. Rubin R. (2018). Exploring the Relationship Between Depression and Dementia. *JAMA*, 320(10), 961–962. https://doi.org/10.1001/jama.2018.11154.

Suicide

15. Barker, J., Oakes-Rogers, S., & Leddy, A. (2022). What distinguishes high and low-lethality suicide attempts in older adults? A systematic review and meta-analysis. *Journal of psychiatric research*, 154, 91–101. https://doi.org/10.1016/j.jpsychires.2022.07.048

16. Beghi, M., Butera, E., Cerri, C. G., Cornaggia, C. M., Febbo, F., Mollica, A., Berardino, G., Piscitelli, D., Resta, E., Logroscino, G., Daniele, A., Altamura, M., Bellomo, A., Panza, F., & Lozupone, M. (2021). Suicidal behaviour in older age: A systematic review of risk factors associated to suicide attempts and completed suicides. *Neuroscience and biobehavioral reviews*, 127, 193–211. https://doi.org/10.1016/j.neubiorev.2021.04.011

17. Chattun, M. R., Amdanee, N., Zhang, X., & Yao, Z. (2022). Suicidality in the geriatric population. *Asian journal of psychiatry*, 75, 103213. https://doi.org/10.1016/j.ajp.2022.103213

18. Cleveland Clinic. "What To Know About Older Adults and Suicide Risk." Mental Health, Cleveland Clinic. 2023, April 4. https://health.clevelandclinic.org/suicide-in-older-adults/#:~:text=Adults%20age%2065%2B%20are%20at,1%20in%204%20older%20adults.

19. Crestani, C., Masotti, V., Corradi, N., Schirripa, M. L., & Cecchi, R. Suicide in the elderly: a 37-year retrospective study. Acta bio-medica : AteneiParmensis, (2019). 90 (1), 68–76. https://doi.org/10.23750/abm.v90i1.6312.

20. Harmer, B., Lee, S., Duong, T., Vi, H., & Saadabadi, A. (2023). *Suicidal ideation*. In StatPearls. StatPearls Publishing. http://www.ncbi.nlm.nih.gov/books/NBK565877/

21. Jamison, K.R. *Night falls fast: Understanding suicide* (1st ed). Knopf. 1999.

22. Motillon-Toudic, C., Walter, M., Séguin M., Carrier J.D., Berrouiguet, S., Lemey, C. *Social isolation and suicide risk: Literature review and perspectives. EurPsychiatry.* 2022 Oct 11;65(1):e65. doi: 10.1192/j.eurpsy.2022.2320. PMID: 36216777; PMCID: PMC9641655.

Chapter 8: Beyond Sadness

1. Bereavement and Grief. (2023). MIA: Mental Health America; Mental Health America. https://www.mhnational.org/bereavement-and-grief.

2. Taylor-Desir, M. "What is Posttraumatic Stress Disorder (PTSD)?" *American Psychiatric Association.* November 2022. http://www.psychiatry.org/patients-families/ptsd/what-is-ptsd?

Chapter 10: Illusions: Some We Need, Some We Don't.

1. Zanto, T.P., & Gazzaley,A.. Aging of the frontal lobe. In *Handbook of Clinical Neurology.* Vol.163, pp. 369-389. 2019. Elsevier. http://doi.org/10.10.1016/B978-0-12-804281-6.00020-3.

2. Fuster, J.M. (2015). *The Prefrontal Cortex.* Academic Press. www. Elsevier.com

Chapter 11: Resilience

1. Milton, J. (n.d.). Sonnet 19: When I consider how my light is spent. *Poems and Poets*; Poetry Foundation. http://www.poetryfoundation.org/poems/47750/sonnet-19-when-i-consider-how-my-light-is-spent.

2. Thomas, D. (2017). *The Poems of Dylan Thomas* (J. Goodby,Ed.). New Directions. http://www.amazon.com/Poems-Dylan-Thomas-/dp/081221148

Chapter 13: Accepting New Roles

1. Ted Lasso Reacts (2021, April 24). "Ted Lasso: Be curious,not judgmental." *YouTube.* http://www.youtube.com/watch?v=i FofLSherM

Chapter 15: So Much Depends On Lunch

1. Blizzard: A type of frozen treat with candy bars mixed in with soft serve ice cream.

Chapter 16: Inner Voices

1. Garrett, L. "Why We Talk to Ourselves: The Science of Your Internal Monologue." Mindful: Healthy Mind, Healthy Life; Mindful Communications & Such. 2022, November 3. https://www.mindful.org/why-we-talk-to-ourselves-the-science-of-your-internal-monologue/

2. *Oxford English Dictionary.* About the OED/Oxford English Dictionary. https://www.oed.com/information/about-the-oed.

Chapter 17: Just Between Us

1. Harari, Y.N. *Sapiens: A brief history of humankind.* First U.S. edition. Harper.

2. Snowdon, David. *Aging with Grace: What the Nun Study Teaches Us about Leading Longer, Healthier, and More Meaningful Lives.* Bantam, 2002.

3. Harvard Study of Human Development. Best place to start is the TEDTalk by Robert Waldiner, the current director.

4. McCann, R.M. "Communication, Aging and Culture." In R.M. McCann, *Oxford Research Encyclopedia of Communication.* Oxford University Press. 2017.

ABOUT the AUTHOR

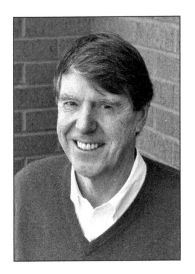

Dr. Charles Edwards practiced cardiovascular surgery for 30 years in his hometown of Charlotte, N.C. Deeply affected by his parent's struggles with dementia, at age 65 he sought further training in dementia which resulted in the founding of Memory and Movement Charlotte in 2013. The care of patients with memory loss and those caring for them has been life changing for Dr. Edwards. This intense experience has been the source of his two books, *Much Abides* and *Late Fragment*.

ABOUT the ARTIST

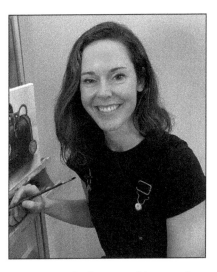

Leslie Edwards is an artist living and working in New York City. She works in the realist tradition in a variety of mediums—mostly oil, watercolor, and pen and ink drawing. Leslie studied at the Art Students League of New York, where her painting was awarded the George A. Rada Memorial Merit Scholarship in 2022. She is a graduate of Middlebury College and earned a Masters in Contemporary Art and Design at Christie's Education in London. She is married with two daughters.

This is her first time illustrating a book. You can find more of her work at www.leslieedwardsstudio.com.

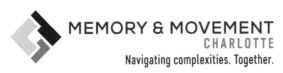

MEMORY & MOVEMENT
CHARLOTTE
Navigating complexities. Together.

Memory & Movement Charlotte
411 Billingsley Road, #103
Charlotte, NC 28211-1066
Phone: (704) 577-3186
Website: www.mmclt.org

A portion of proceeds from book sales support Memory & Movement Charlotte. The 501c(3) clinic provides medical care, education, and support to individuals with memory and movement disorders and their caregivers.

Appointments involve a multi-disciplinary, physician-led team and last 60 to 90 minutes. Services include monthly education sessions, onsite therapeutic gym, podcasts, support programs and online library. Educational resources are freely available.

Since 2013, it has experienced steady growth. In the last fiscal year, 1,366 patients and 3,415 caregivers were served. Support comprehensive, family-centric care and learn more at

www.mmclt.org

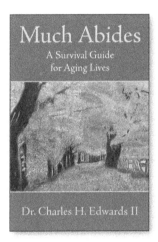 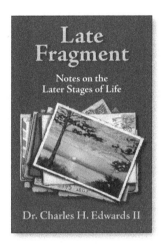

Dr. Edwards' first book, *Much Abides: A Survival Guide for Aging Lives*, helps seniors find passion and purpose in their post-retirement years. It offers encouragement and practical advice on how to embrace this chapter in your life story.

Much Abides and *Late Fragment* are for sale at Memory & Movement Charlotte (www.mmclt.org), Park Road Books (www.parkroadbooks.com) in Charlotte, N.C., and online at www.amazon.com and other booksellers. Cost for each is $25.

Sales support Memory & Movement Charlotte.

Printed in the USA
CPSIA information can be obtained
at www.ICGtesting.com
LVHW050458221123
764280LV00008B/20